Breast Disease for Radiographers

Jennifer Caseldine, Roger Blamey, Eric Roebuck and Christopher Elston
Nottingham City Hospital, Nottingham

WRIGHT

London   Boston   Singapore   Sydney   Toronto   Wellington

John Wright
is an imprint of Butterworth Scientific

First published, 1988

© **Butterworth & co. (Publishers) Ltd, 1988**

British Library Cataloguing in Publication Data

Breast disease for radiographers.
  1. Women. Breasts. Diseases
  I. Caseldine, Jennifer
  618.1′9

  ISBN 0-7236-1067-3

Library of Congress Cataloging in Publication Data

Breast disease for radiographers / Jennifer Caseldine . . . [et al.].
    p. cm.
  Includes index.
  ISBN 0-7236-1067-3:
  1. Breast--Cancer--Diagnosis. 2. Breast--Radiography. 3. Breast-
-Diseases--Diagnosis. I. Caseldine, Jennifer.
  [DNLM: 1. Breast Diseases--diagnosis. 2. Breast Diseases-
-therapy. 3. Breast Neoplasms--radiography. 4. Breast Neoplasms-
-therapy. 5. Mammography. WP 840 B8285]
RC280.B8B7145 1988
618.1′90757--dc19
DNLM/DLC   88-11632
for Library of Congress   CIP

Photoset by Butterworths Litho Preparation Department
Printed and bound by Hartnolls Ltd, Bodmin, Cornwall

The authors

Acknowledgements

Jennifer Caseldine is Superintendent Radiographer in charge of the Helen Garrod Breast Screening Unit at Nottingham City Hospital and Research Fellow in Breast Cancer in the Professorial Unit of Surgery. Since 1979 she has been responsible for the programme of education for breast self-examination and for the clinical and mammographic assessment of women subsequently self-referring and for the mammographic service for symptomatic women.

Roger Blamey is Professor of Surgical Science at Nottingham City Hospital. He is in clinical charge of perhaps the largest programme for breast disease in the country. The Nottingham City Hospital breast team has published widely on research and clinical work in breast cancer. He is a member of the British Breast Group.

Eric Roebuck is Consultant Radiologist at the Nottingham Hospitals. He was a member of the 'Forrest' committee of the Department of Health which reported on breast cancer screening and is a member of the European Group for Breast Cancer Screening and the British Breast Group and is Registrar of the Royal College of Radiologists.

Christopher Elston is Consultant Pathologist at Nottingham City Hospital and is responsible for the histological aspects of the clinical and research programme at the City Hospital. He is a member of the Committee for Clinical Trials in Breast Cancer and of the British Breast Group.

We wish to thank Wendy Bartlam for the transcription of the manuscript, Keith Gordon for photomicrography, Stella Winfield, Verdi Stickland, Anne Rose, Toni Bain and Patricia Walker for their work in the Helen Garrod Breast Screening Unit from where the mammograms were taken, Geoffrey Gilbert for the photography and John Robertson, Adrian Locker and Anna Mitchell for their help in analyses and presentation of our results.

Contents

Introduction

The investigation of breast disease involves diagnostic radiographers in many ways. The radiographer deals with screening of asymptomatic patients, investigation of breast lumps, follow-up after treating a primary cancer, the investigation of secondary spread and the assessment of response to treatment. The first of these, screening, is in the process of being expanded to cover every woman in the country in her lifetime so that many more radiographers will be needed in this field.

It is the belief of the authors that radiographers should be involved at an interesting and responsible level and not simply act as 'button pressers'. Specialized knowledge of the disease they investigate allows them to become part of the breast cancer team. In Nottingham, for the last 7 years, a programme of education for breast self-examination for self-referral has been in progress. At the Helen Garrod Breast Screening Unit the radiographers carry out the majority of this programme themselves: they give the education lectures (*Figure 1*), examine clinically those patients who return to the Unit with a breast problem and make a decision as to whether the breast is normal or abnormal, take a mammogram and carry out the first reading of this. They use ultrasound in a real-time situation to decide if mammographic opacities denote a cyst. Women showing no abnormality either clinically or mammographically are reassured and are not seen by any medically qualified staff. The system has worked well and some 5000 women presenting back to the unit symptomatically have been able to

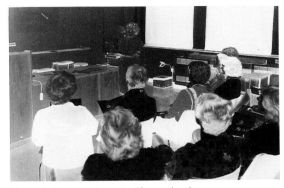

Figure 1 A talk on breast self-examination

receive rapid assessment and reassurance in this way in Nottingham. Our radiographers have taken clinical decisions and have enjoyed the responsibilities which were additional to their role in producing mammograms of the highest quality.

The book leans towards early detection and mammography and this is inevitably so in view of the introduction of the national screening programme. The Helen Garrod Unit at Nottingham City Hospital is a designated training unit with programmes for screening and mammographic technique, mammographic basic screen reading and training for clinical examination and lecturing for breast self-examination. The programme for screening and mammographic technique includes all aspects approved by a committee established by the College of Radiographers (*see* Appendix).

1

Breast cancer – aetiology and prognosis

Breast cancer is the commonest malignancy in women. Twenty-six thousand new cases are diagnosed in the UK and 15 000 women die from the disease each year.

Aetiology

The only aetiological factor of strength within the population of this country is family history, i.e.

mother, maternal grandmother or sister with breast cancer. Around 15 per cent of breast cancers have such a history. Occasional families are seen with a very high incidence of breast cancer and such occurrence argues the case for a genetic predisposition. A genetic factor may expose women to causative influences and hormonal and dietary factors have been cited.

The evidence for these factors is indirect. Japanese women have a lower incidence of breast

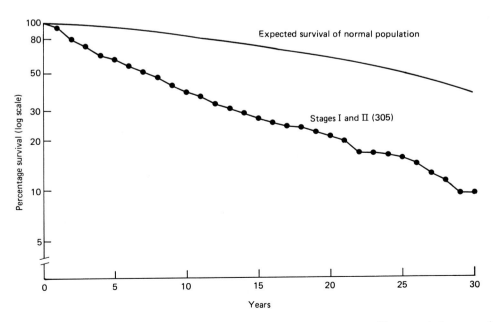

Figure 1.1 Graphs of survival of 305 cases of stage I and II breast cancer over a 35-year period compared with that of age-matched women without breast cancer. (By kind permission of Dr John Haybittle)

cancer than Western women, but the incidence rises in 'Westernized' Japanese; this argues for Western lifestyle-linked factors which possibly lie in the diet. Premenopausal women who have undergone oophorectomy have a degree of protection against breast cancer, and late menarche and early first pregnancy also have a protective effect; these argue for a hormonally linked causative factor.

Prognosis

Once a woman develops breast cancer, what is the outlook? The study by John Haybittle and Diana Brinkley followed 704 cases of breast cancer over a 30- to 35-year period. The survival graph is seen in *Figure 1.1* where the survival curves are seen of the cases of early breast cancer, i.e. cases staged I and II (tumours that measured less than 5 cm and without skin fixity) and the expected survival of an age-matched population of women without breast cancer.

At 20–25 years from diagnosis, taking only the patients with the 'early' cancers, only 20–25 per cent are still alive. The expected survival at this time of the non-breast-cancerous population is 75 per cent. In other words, at 25 years from diagnosis of breast cancer one patient out of five is still alive, one has died of causes other than breast cancer and three have died of breast cancer.

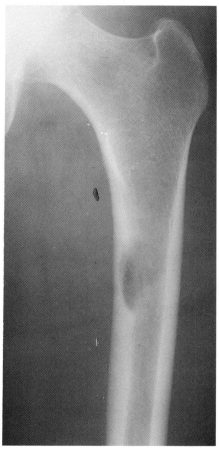

Figure 1.2 X-ray of femur showing an area of bone destruction due to a secondary deposit

Metastatic spread

The primary growth in the breast does not kill the women. It is the distant spread to other organs via the bloodstream from the primary growth that kills. This spread is therefore present in at least three out of five women at the time their tumour is diagnosed.

Metastatic spread in breast cancer is most commonly to bones (*Figure 1.2*), liver, lung and pleura (*Figure 1.3*). It may also be seen in the brain or spinal cord, peritoneal cavity, bone marrow, ovaries and skin.

Once distant spread has become recognized from symptoms such as bone pain or breathlessness, death from breast cancer is inevitable. Fifty per cent of patients showing symptoms from distant spread will die within 1 year of the appearance of these symptoms (*Figure 1.4*).

Prognosis in the individual case

Once breast cancer has presented, what factors will influence whether the woman will die of her disease in a few years, at 20 years or will survive her breast cancer?

The size at which a cancer is diagnosed is important: as might be expected, the smaller the tumour the more likely is long-term survival. This is the logical basis for screening for breast cancer which is discussed in detail in Chapters 11 and 12.

Invasion by cancer of the lymph nodes draining the breast means that the cancer has spread to other organs. The lymphatics are not currently considered to be the main route of spread (which is the bloodstream) but lymphatic invasion correlates with

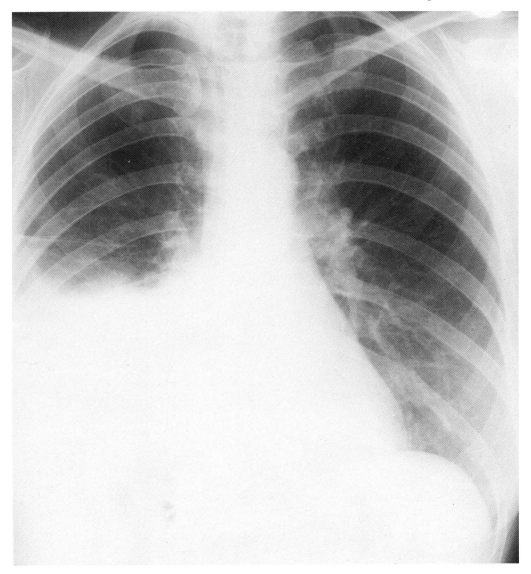

Figure 1.3 Chest X-ray showing a pleural effusion due to secondary deposits on the surface of the lung

bloodstream spread and, therefore, acts as an indicator of such spread. The influence of lymphatic spread on survival is seen in *Figure 1.5.*

The routes of lymphatic spread from the breast are to the axillary nodes and to the internal mammary nodes lying behind the costal cartilages just beside the sternum.

Size of the primary and stage of lymphatic invasion are two prognostic factors dependent upon time: the longer the tumour has been there the more advanced they will be. However, the biological nature (the speed of growth, sensitivity to hormones etc.) of the tumour may change only slightly once it is established and is the same in the primary tumour as in the distant metastases. These properties of a biological nature are best seen as the histological grade, i.e. whether the cells of a tumour are not too dissimilar to those of the normal breast (well differentiated; *Figure 1.6*) or whether they are wildly different with numerous abnormal and

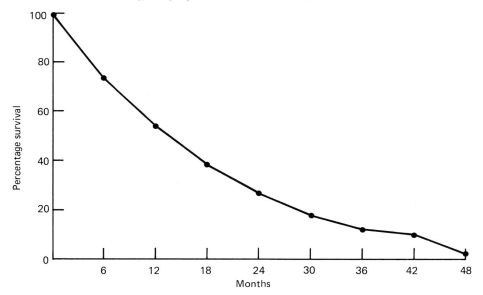

Figure 1.4 Graph of survival of 190 women with secondary breast cancer (stage IV) from the time that the distant spread gave symptoms

multiplying cells (*Figure 1.7*; poorly differentiated). The effect of histological grade on survival is seen in *Figure 1.8*.

Combining these factors of size, stage and grade, it is possible to get a good idea of the chance of an individual patient developing distant spread and dying or remaining free from breast cancer (*Figure 1.9*).

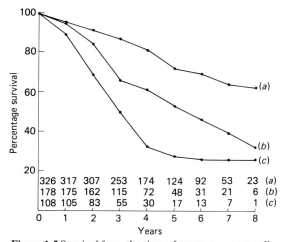

Figure 1.5 Survival from the time of mastectomy according to whether lymph nodes around the breast were free of cancer (*a*), or involved: (*b*) low axilla involved; (*c*) high node involvement. $\chi^2 = 246.3$; two degrees of freedom; $P < 0.0005$

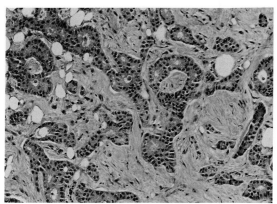

Figure 1.6 Well-differentiated carcinoma. the cells are arranged in clear tubules and nuclei are regular. Haematoxylin and eosin, ×114

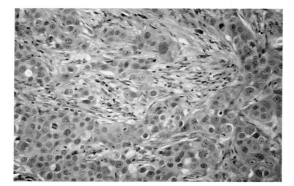

Figure 1.7 Poorly differentiated carcinoma. There is no tubule formation, marked pleomorphism and several mitoses are present. Haematoxylin and eosin, ×143

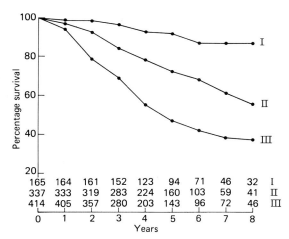

Figure 1.8 The effect of histological differentiation on survival from the time of mastectomy: I, well differentiated; II, moderate; III, poor differentiation. $\chi^2 = 90.86$; two degrees of freedom; $P<0.0005$

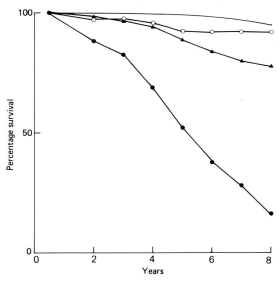

Figure 1.9 Survival from the time of mastectomy according to the Nottingham prognostic index. The index depends upon a combination of tumour size, stage and grade. ○—○, Tumours with good index; ▲—▲ those with moderate index; ●—● those with poor index. At 10 years, 85 per cent of the good index patients are alive, but only 5 per cent of the poor index patients. Comparison with the survival of age-matched women without breast cancer (——) is shown

2

The histopathology of breast disease

The normal breast

The breasts are modified apocrine sweat glands. Before puberty the structure of male and female breast tissue is identical, consisting of a rudimentary branching duct system which discharges onto the surface at the nipple. At puberty, under the influence of oestrogenic stimulation, the female breast enlarges due both to an increase in the amount of stromal connective and adipose tissue and to a proliferation of the duct system. Breast lobules composed of acini and intralobular stroma bud from subsegmental ducts to form physiologically functional, terminal duct lobular units (*Figure 2.1*). Microscopically, the ducts and acini are lined by an inner secretory epithelial cell and an outer

myoepithelial cell within the basement membrane (*Figure 2.2*).

During pregnancy the lobules enlarge due to an increase in the size and number of acini. Secretory activity increases within the epithelial cells and luminal secretions appear. At the onset of lactation, secretory activity becomes more pronounced with a large distension of acini and relative obliteration of connective tissue.

Following pregnancy and lactation, involutional changes occur in the lobules as they return to the resting state. Involutional changes also occur with age, especially postmenopausally. Lobules become atrophic due to a contraction in the size of acini and hyalinization of intralobular stroma.

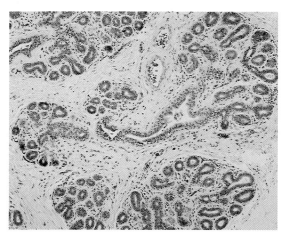

Figure 2.1 Normal breast tissue from a young nulliparous female. A complete terminal duct lobular unit is seen at the top right. Haematoxylin and eosin, ×66

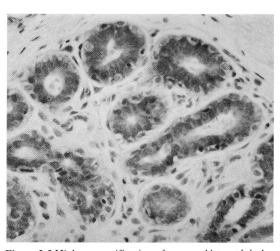

Figure 2.2 Higher magnification of a normal breast lobule. Note the two cell types which line the acini. Haematoxylin and eosin, ×264

Developmental abnormalities

Congenital abnormalities of the breast are rare and unimportant with the exception of polymastia and polythelia – accessory nipples. These may occur anywhere along the 'milk line' and are subject to the same disorders as normally situated breasts.

Failure of development of the breasts at puberty is very uncommon and usually associated with ovarian agenesis, as in Turner's syndrome. Precocious development may also occur, occasionally related to the presence of an ovarian granulosa cell tumour, but usually for unexplained reasons.

Adolescent or juvenile hypertrophy is the commonest developmental abnormality found. At the onset of puberty the breasts grow rapidly and out of proportion, so that they become a severe physical and psychological burden. Rarely, the hypertrophy is unilateral. The cause is unknown and the only effective treatment is surgical reduction. Microscopically, no specific abnormality is seen and the enlargement appears to be due to an overgrowth of adipose and connective tissue.

Benign breast lesions

The term 'benign breast disease' is often used clinically to imply a specific pathological entity. This is clearly an oversimplification and there are a number of distinct lesions which merit discussion.

Fibrocystic change

A very wide range of terms is used synonymously for this condition including fibroadenosis, cystic hyperplasia, chronic mastitis and mammary dysplasia. None is entirely satisfactory but fibrocystic change has become the most widely accepted. The condition is the commonest of all breast lesions, and produces clinical symptoms in at least 10 per cent of women. It usually presents as a discrete lump in the breast or as a more general 'lumpiness' which occasionally may be bilateral. The peak frequency is in the premenopausal decade and after the menopause there is a sharp decline in symptomatic cases. As breast screening becomes more widespread, an increasing number of cases will be detected mammographically.

The underlying cause of fibrocystic change is not well understood. The lesion is not part of an inflammatory process, as some of the terms imply, but almost certainly has a hormonal basis. The cyclical activity of the ovary, with alternating oestrogen and progesterone secretion, produces changes in the breasts as well as the endometrium. Subtle proliferative changes occur in the breast lobules during the menstrual cycle and it is likely that these become exaggerated and abnormal in the premenopausal era due to hormonal imbalance related to diminishing ovarian function. Histologically, a range of appearances may be seen, and the microscopical components described below are present in variable amounts from case to case.

Cystic change

It is the presence of cysts (*Figure 2.3*) which most frequently produces clinical symptoms in the form of a palpable lump. They may be simple or multiple and usually contain clear fluid. Cysts are derived

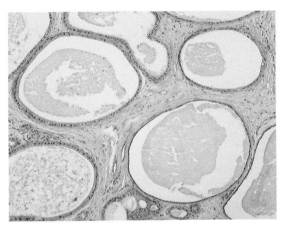

Figure 2.3 Fibrocystic change: in this field a number of fluid-filled cystic structures is shown. Haematoxylin and eosin, ×66

from lobular acini and are frequently only detectable microscopically as so-called 'microcysts'. They are lined by flattened epithelium, and the wall is often thickened due to reactive inflammation and fibrosis.

Epithelial proliferation

Frequently, the epithelial lining of lobular acini and cysts undergoes metaplasia to columnar cells resembling those of normal apocrine sweat glands, the so-called pink cell change or apocrine metaplasia (*Figure 2.4*). The degree of proliferation varies but papillary structures may be seen.

In about a quarter of cases a significant degree of epithelial proliferation is seen within ductular structures. In Europe, this process is usually

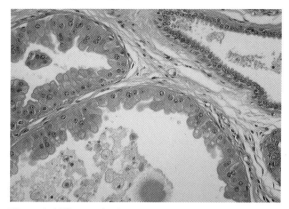

Figure 2.4 Fibrocystic change: the cells lining the ducts on the left have undergone apocrine metaplasia. Haematoxylin and eosin, ×156

referred to as epitheliosis, but in the USA the term 'papillomatosis' is used. The lumen of the ductules is lined by several layers of large epithelial cells having abundant cytoplasm (*Figures 2.5* and *2.6*), and the lumen may be obliterated by a solid proliferation. The cells often have an organized 'streaming' pattern especially when ducts are dilated by a florid proliferation. Nuclei are regular in appearance and, although occasional mitoses are seen, they are not of normal configuration. Cell necrosis is not seen.

In cases where abnormal features are present in an epithelial proliferation, considerable diagnostic difficulty may be encountered in distinguishing a benign lesion from carcinoma *in situ*. For this borderline category of atypical epithelial hyperpla-

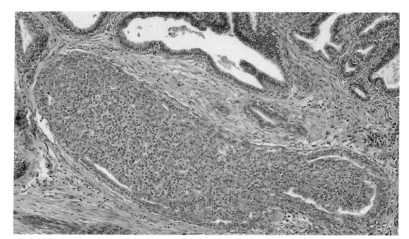

Figure 2.5 Fibrocystic change: the lumen of the duct is filled with a regular proliferation of benign epithelial cells (epitheliosis). Haematoxylin and eosin, ×77

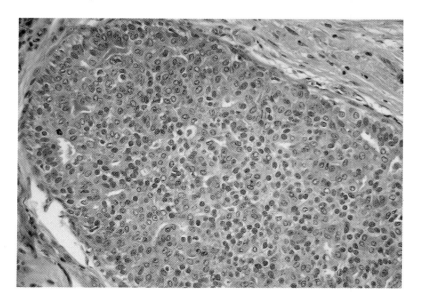

Figure 2.6 Higher magnification of *Figure 2.5*, showing a 'streaming' pattern with regular nuclei. Haematoxylin and eosin, ×208

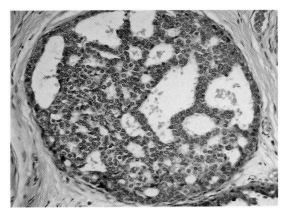

Figure 2.7 Atypical ductal hyperplasia: the epithelial proliferation forms an irregular lacy network, but there is no nuclear pleomorphism. Haematoxylin and eosin, ×156

sia, Page and colleagues have adopted a very simple and broad definition; they use the term to categorize those lesions which have some, but not all, of the morphological and cytological features of *in situ* malignancy. Two types of atypical hyperplasia are recognized: ductal and lobular. In atypical ductal hyperplasia, the commonest pattern is that of an irregular lacy network resembling cribriform ductal carcinoma *in situ*, but lacking the necessary rigid geometric configuration (compare *Figure 2.7* with *Figure 2.15*). A micropapillary pattern may also be seen. Mitoses and nuclear hyperchromatism are present in variable degrees; cellular necrosis of 'comedo' type is absent.

In atypical lobular hyperplasia, although definite epithelial proliferation occurs there is little or no increase in the size of lobules and only minimal expansion of acini. There may be partial involvement of lobules and most acinar lumina are preserved (compare *Figure 2.8* with *Figure 2.16*).

Adenosis

The broad terms 'adenosis' and 'fibroadenosis' are greatly over-used by pathologists, often when no abnormality is present, and should be abandoned. In blunt-duct adenosis there is an organoid hypertrophy of lobules with dilatation of acini and an increase in intralobular stroma. The term 'sclerosing adenosis' denotes a specific proliferative lesion of the terminal duct lobular unit. There are two main types: multifocal, which is a component of fibrocystic change, and nodular, which may occur as a tumour-like mass in an otherwise normal breast, especially in younger women. Microscopically the normal configuration of lobules is distorted by a disorderly proliferation of epithelial, myoepithelial and intralobular stromal cells (*Figure 2.9*). A whorled pattern of microtubules may be seen but luminal structures are often indistinct. The nuclei are of regular appearance without atypia and mitoses are infrequent.

Fine speckled microcalcification is usually present (*Figure 2.10*) but may be scanty. In the uncommon variant of sclerosing adenosis, microglandular adenosis, microtubular structures may be present within adipose tissue, the appearances mimicking an infiltrating carcinoma (*Figure 2.11*).

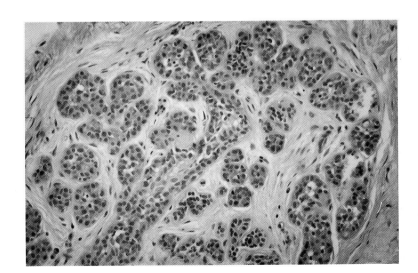

Figure 2.8 Atypical lobular hyperplasia: there is proliferation of epithelial cells within acini but clear lumina are preserved. Haematoxylin and eosin, ×195

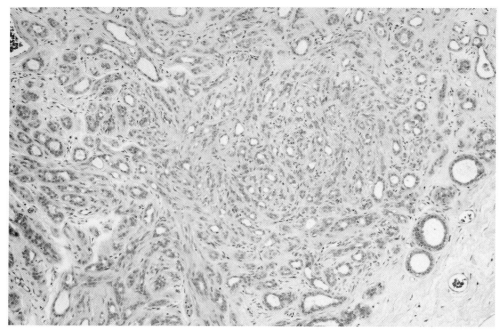

Figure 2.9 Sclerosing adenosis: lobules are distorted by a disorderly cellular proliferation. Haematoxylin and eosin, ×70

Radial scar

A varied and confusing nomenclature has been applied to this distinctive sclerosing lesion of the breast including 'sclerosing papillary proliferation' and 'infiltrating epitheliosis', but 'radial scar' has emerged as the preferred term. Morphologically, it is composed of a nodule of radiating stellate connective tissue with a dense fibroelastic core (*Figure 2.12*). It varies from 5 to 10 mm in diameter.

Within the arms of the stellate configuration ductules appear to be drawn into the centre, and a variable degree of epithelial proliferation is seen.

Radial scars were once thought to be uncommon, but with the greater use of mammography, they are known to occur relatively frequently. The precise pathogenesis is uncertain, but most evidence suggests that radial scars form part of the spectrum of fibrocystic change.

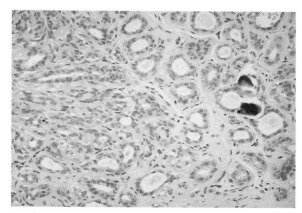

Figure 2.10 Higher magnification of sclerosing adenosis to show a focus of microcalcification to the right. Haematoxylin and eosin, ×156

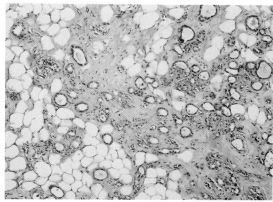

Figure 2.11 Microglandular adenosis: note the apparent infiltration of adipose tissue by microtubular structures. Haematoxylin and eosin, ×66

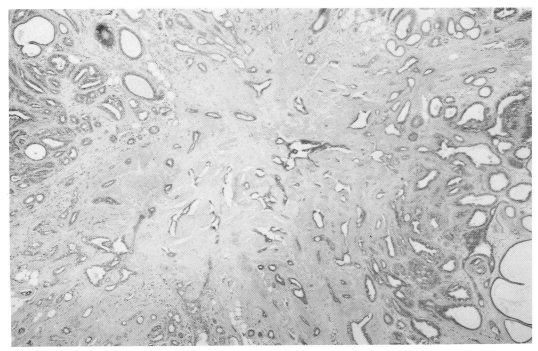

Figure 2.12 Radial scar: low power view of the central portion. Haematoxylin and eosin, ×40

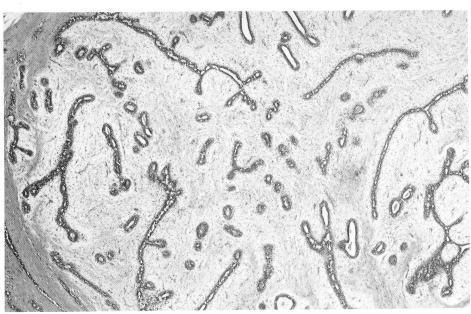

Figure 2.13 Fibroadenoma: the abundant stroma and epithelial clefts are clearly defined. Haematoxylin and eosin, ×40

Fibroadenoma

Although it has been conventional to classify fibroadenomas as benign tumours, there is considerable evidence to support the view that they are not true neoplasms but focal areas of lobular hyperplasia caused predominantly by an overgrowth of intralobular stroma. They may present at any age after puberty, but are most common under 30 years. Clinically they appear as small, firm, well-defined mobile lumps in the breast which are occasionally multiple.

Histologically, they are composed of proliferating ductules and stroma with characteristic cleft-like spaces and periacinar whorls (*Figure 2.13*). They are circumscribed but not encapsulated.

Papilloma

Intraduct papillomas are uncommon benign neoplasms, occuring predominantly in middle-aged patients. The presenting symptom in the majority of cases is single duct discharge from the nipple; the discharge may be bloodstained. They are usually single and located in one of the main ducts near the nipple. Microscopically, they consist of a fronded fibrovascular core covered by a two-layered duct-type epithelium. Occasionally, the duct becomes cystically dilated thus forming an intracystic papilloma; this may present as a palpable nodule.

The great majority of ductal papillomas pursue a benign course. In rare cases papillomas may be multiple and these usually involve smaller ducts. In such cases there appears to be an increased risk of subsequent carcinoma.

Benign breast disease and risk of malignancy

Since it was first suggested over 40 years ago that patients with fibrocystic change have an increased risk of developing a subsequent breast carcinoma, the subject has been the centre of much controversy. Many of the studies performed have had serious methodological flaws and it is only recently that a degree of clarity has been achieved by the work of Page and colleagues. They have shown that patients whose biopsies show no epithelial hyperplasia have no increased risk; because this category accounts for approximately 70 per cent of all non-malignant biopsies, the great majority of women can be reassured and do not require follow-up. The presence of regular epithelial hyperplasia increases the risk of subsequent carcinoma two-fold, and these biopsies amount to 25 per cent of the total. The most sigificant increase in risk (of four times) occurs in patients whose biopsies show atypical epithelial hyperplasia, and this is doubled in the presence of a family history of breast cancer. However, epithelial atypia is found in only 4 per cent of biopsies and atypia with a family history in 1 per cent. Long-term follow-up is advisable for the very small group of patients with epithelial atypia; they should be taught breast self-examination and offered yearly mammography. Unfortunately, these histological criteria are of little value in identifying high-risk groups for screening purposes because so few patients are selected.

Furthermore, the data need to be put in perspective. In the highest risk group, i.e. epithelial atypia with family history, only 20 per cent of the patients actually developed an invasive carcinoma within the succeeding 15 years. The great majority remained tumour free, which emphasizes the need for therapeutic caution. It is interesting to note that only one patient in 50 who presents with breast cancer has ever had previous breast surgery.

Carcinoma of the breast

Carcinoma of the breast is still the commonest malignant tumour in women, although now it is closely followed by carcinoma of the bronchus. The frequency appears to be increasing, especially in younger women, and this is not entirely due to an increase in the 'at risk' population. It may occur at any age, but is rare below the age of 25 years and most frequent between 40 and 70 years.

Despite the identification of a number of risk factors, the aetiology of breast cancer remains obscure. A positive family history increases the risk significantly, but is present in a very small group of patients. As noted above, women whose breast biopsy shows epithelial proliferation are also at increased risk, but this too identifies a minority of patients. There is slight protection when the first child is born early in the reproductive age span, and also from late menarche and early menopause. No consistent hormonal abnormalities have been associated with breast cancer, nor are there convincing data that exogenous oestrogen therapy is a risk factor. Experimental work in mice has shown that an RNA virus is the main aetiological agent, but to date there is no evidence to implicate a virus in human breast cancer.

In the majority of cases carcinoma of the breast presents as a single palpable lump. This may occur anywhere in the breast, but the upper outer quadrant is the commonest site. It is hoped that with the introduction of breast screening an increasing number of impalpable tumours will be detected mammographically.

Carcinoma of the breast is subdivided pathologically into two broad categories: *in situ* and invasive carcinoma.

In situ carcinoma

By definition, in an *in situ* carcinoma the cytological changes of malignancy are present in the epithelial cells of an organ or structure, but the basement membrane is intact and no evidence of stromal invasion is seen. In the breast two types of carcinoma *in situ* are recognized: ductal and lobular.

Ductal carcinoma *in situ*

A variable number of ducts or ductular structures is involved. They contain a proliferation of large epithelial cells with abundant cytoplasm, a variable degree of nuclear pleomorphism and increased mitoses. The epithelial proliferations may be solid, often with central necrosis (comedo carcinoma) (*Figure 2.14*), have the appearance of a lacy network (cribriform type) (*Figure 2.15*) or have a micropapillary pattern. The basement membrane may be thickened but remains intact.

In Paget's disease of the nipple, which presents as a red, scaly, eczematous lesion involving the nipple and areola, there is always an underlying ductal carcinoma *in situ*. This is usually impalpable, and may be situated deep in the breast tissue or confined to large nipple ducts. The eczematous rash appears to be due to permeation of the nipple epithelium by carcinoma cells which migrate up the ducts into the epidermis.

Lobular carcinoma *in situ*

This type is characterized by the proliferation of small epithelial cells within the acini of a group of lobules, obliterating the acinar lumen. The lobular units are distended and the intralobular stroma relatively reduced. Basement membranes remain intact (*Figure 2.16*).

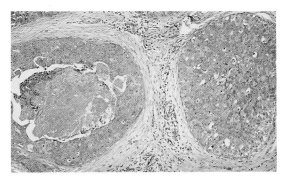

Figure 2.14 Ductal carcinoma *in situ*, of the solid type. Note the central luminal necrosis in the ductule on the left. Haematoxylin and eosin, ×52

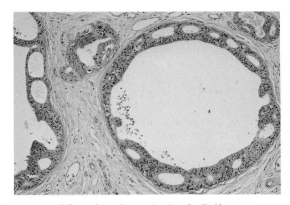

Figure 2.15 Ductal carcinoma *in situ* of cribriform type. Haematoxylin and eosin, ×57

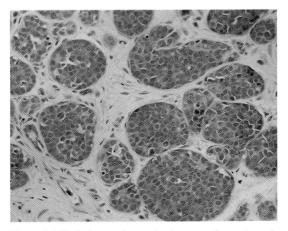

Figure 2.16 Lobular carcinoma *in situ*: part of an enlarged lobule in which the acini are distended by a solid proliferation of small epithelial cells. Haematoxylin and eosin, ×170

Invasive carcinoma

Invasive carcinoma of the breast arises from a pre-existing *in situ* carcinoma, although by the time the tumour has presented clinically the *in situ* element may no longer be detectable histologically. The following main histological types are recognized.

Ductal

Over 50 per cent of invasive breast carcinomas are composed of sheets and cords of large epithelial cells which infiltrate the connective tissue stroma and have no special morphological features (*Figure 2.17*).

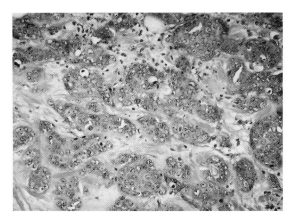

Figure 2.17 Infiltrating ductal carcinoma: cords of tumour cells are seen invading into the adjacent stroma. Haematoxylin and eosin, ×156

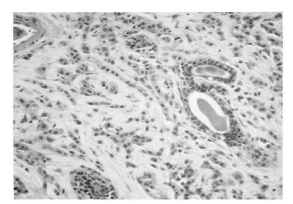

Figure 2.18 Infiltrating lobular carcinoma: single cords of monotonous tumour cells infiltrate the stroma. Note the preserved normal ductules at the right. Haematoxylin and eosin, ×158

Infiltrating lobular

This is the invasive counterpart of lobular carcinoma *in situ* and accounts for about 10 per cent of invasive carcinomas. Classically, linear cords of small epithelial cells infiltrate diffusely within connective tissue giving a so-called 'Indian file' pattern (*Figure 2.18*). The infiltrate often assumes a concentric 'targetoid' arrangement around preserved normal structures.

Medullary carcinoma

These rare tumours have a well circumscribed edge and are composed of anastomosing sheets of epithelial cells forming syncytial masses, with a conspicuous lymphoplasmacytoid infiltrate in the stroma (*Figure 2.19*). No tubule formation is seen and the epithelial cells have a poorly differentiated appearance with a high mitotic rate.

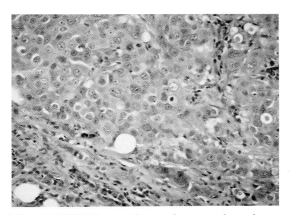

Figure 2.19 Medullary carcinoma: the tumour has a sharp edge, with a conspicuous lymphoplasmacytic infiltrate. Haematoxylin and eosin, ×156

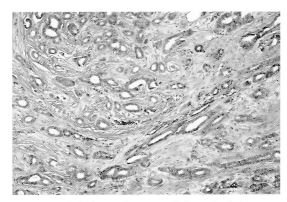

Figure 2.20 Tubular carcinoma: well-formed tubules infiltrate a cellular stroma. Haematoxylin and eosin, ×116

Tubular carcinoma

Tubular carcinomas are tumours composed of small uniform epithelial cells arranged in well-defined tubular structures (*Figure 2.20*). They are small (usually less than 1 cm in diameter), firm and have an irregular stellate outline. The tubules are lined by a single layer of regular epithelial cells and lumina are patent. Mitoses are rarely seen. The stroma is cellular and the centre of the tumour is frequently elastotic.

Pure tubular carcinomas are uncommon even using the criterion that 75 per cent rather than 90 per cent of the structure should be tubular. More frequently, tumours are seen in which a tubular element is preserved centrally but at the periphery infiltrating ductal or infiltrating lobular carcinoma occupies more than 25 per cent of the tumour tissue. Such tumours may be designated tubular mixed or tubular variant carcinomas.

Mucoid

These are also known as colloid or mucinous carcinomas. They are uncommon tumours which have a characteristic pale soft gelatinous appearance macroscopically. They are usually well circum-scribed and may become large, even exceeding 5 cm in diameter. Histologically, the tumour is composed of clumps and nests of well differentiated epithelial cells lying in lakes of mucin.

Papillary

These are rare tumours, accounting for less than 1 per cent of breast carcinomas. Although there may occasionally be evidence of an origin from a pre-existing duct or cyst papilloma, in most cases this is not so. Microscopically, there are papillary structures with fibrovascular cores; nuclear differentiation is variable.

Routes of spread

There are three main ways in which breast cancer may spread from the primary site: local, lymphatic and blood.

Local

If the tumour remains undetected it will continue to grow and may eventually invade the overlying skin or the deep muscle and chest wall. This is termed a 'locally advanced primary'.

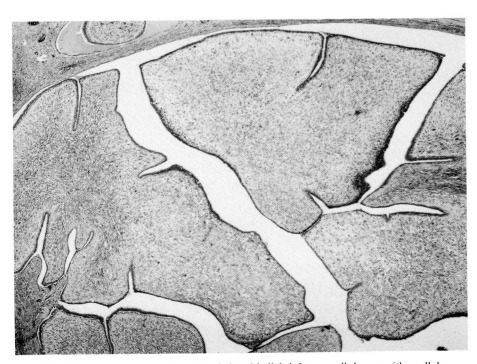

Figure 2.21 Phyllodes tumour: the characteristic epithelial clefts are well shown, with a cellular stroma. Haematoxylin and eosin, ×38

Lymphatic

Dissection studies have shown that the axillary lymph nodes are involved histologically in approximately 50 per cent of patients with apparently 'operable' breast cancer. Lymph node metastasis may also be found in the internal mammary nodes, especially if the primary tumour is located in the inner quadrants. Careful examination of the breast tissue at the periphery of the primary tumour reveals lymphatic permeation in up to 30 per cent of cases.

Blood

This is the route through which distant metastases occur. Unfortunately, three out of four women with breast cancer have bloodstream spread at the time of diagnosis (*see* Chapter 1). Many organs may be involved, but the commonest sites are lung, bone and liver.

Miscellaneous tumours

Phyllodes tumour

These are uncommon and unusual tumours which are still erroneously termed 'giant fibroadenoma' or 'cystosarcoma phyllodes' by some authors. They occur predominantly in middle-aged or elderly females and are only rarely seen below the age of 40 years. They form large lobulated circumscribed masses and may grow rapidly to cause unilateral breast enlargement and, rarely, skin ulceration.

Macroscopically they have a whorled cut surface which resembles a compressed leaf bud (*phyllos* = leaf, Greek) with visible clefts and occasionally cystic spaces (*see Figure 13.4*). Microscopically elonged cleft-like spaces are lined by epithelial cells and there is a cellular stroma (*Figure 2.21*). The epithelial cells are regular and benign, but nuclear abnormalities may be present in the stromal cells and a variable number of mitoses is present. The great majority of phyllodes tumours are benign and complete excision is curative. Approximately 10 per cent will recur locally after enucleation due to incomplete excision and, in less than 5 per cent, true malignant sarcomatous change occurs in the stromal cells.

Sarcomas

Liposarcoma, angiosarcoma and malignant fibrous histiocytomas occur in the breast but are exceedingly rare.

3

Symptoms and signs of breast disease

The commonest reasons for women to present in the breast clinic are a lump and breast pain. Other presentations include nipple discharge, visible breast deformity and axillary node enlargement. *Table 3.1* shows the numbers of patients according to their presenting complaint, sent by their GPs to our referral clinic during 1979.

When a patient complains of a breast lump the history is relatively unimportant. Either she is correct and has a lump requiring investigation or she does not and this can only be resolved by clinical examination.

Several questions should be asked: whether the lump is extremely tender or was tender, red and hot at presentation – this would indicate an abscess. The family history of breast cancer is explored (only that of mother, grandmother or sister); a mother with bilateral breast cancer before the menopause, and/or more than one of these first-degree relatives with breast cancer, are particularly significant histories. When told that a relative had breast cancer, it is often best to enquire when 'she had her mastectomy', because the general public often confuse any cancer with breast cancer.

A past history of breast disease is enquired into; this is taken as being that of a lump which required aspiration or operation.

When the patient complains of breast pain a longer history is required. It is necessary to gauge the severity of the pain and also to classify the type of pain. The severity of the pain is assessed by asking how much difference the pain and tenderness makes to the patient's life – does it stop her working, wake her up, affect her sex life? Many patients will admit that the pain is not too bad, but that they attended their GP to make sure nothing serious was causing the pain. Women often believe that a cancerous breast lump will be painful. This is not so and breast cancer rarely presents as breast pain.

Various types of breast pain are recognized according to the symptoms. The most common is cyclical pain. This is a more extreme variant of the discomfort felt by many women in the premenstrual week. The pain may be bad enough to interfere with the patient's way of life; it is only relieved during the menstrual period, recurring a week later and reaching a peak again in the premenstrual week. The breasts may become very lumpy and tender. This pain is clearly hormonally related.

Another type of breast pain is not cyclical: it is felt on the lateral side of the breast and radiates to the arm. On questioning the patient often admits to pain over the shoulder and paraesthesiae ('pins and needles') in the forearm and hand. This pain is due to pressure on the lower cervical and upper thoracic

Table 3.1 The presenting complaints of patients attending the referral breast clinic in 1979

Main reason for presentation	Nos
Lump in breast	993
Tender 'lumpy' area	110
Breast pain	224
Nipple discharge	75
Nipple retraction	36
Nipple eczema	3
Swelling of breast	7
Others	57
Total	1445

nerve roots as they come from the arm and enter the spine – due to cervical spondylitis (*Figure 3.1*).

A skin deformity (*Figure 3.2*) caused by tether from an underlying lump is a presentation becoming more commonplace now that women have been made aware of breast self-examination. If a lump shows tether then it is almost certainly a carcinoma.

Nipple indrawing may be due to a cancer under the nipple, in which case the whole of the nipple and areola become pulled in (*Figure 3.2*) or to inflammation and shortening of ducts under the nipple. This latter gives a different picture with the centre of the nipple itself pulled in, often in a 'smile' across the nipple (*Figure 3.3*) and this in-pulling is usually correctable by flattening the centre of the nipple on either side.

Nipple discharge (in the absence of a palpable lump) may come from several ducts in both breasts, in which case this is due to a general oversecretion and not a single lesion, or from a single duct. Single duct discharge with no palpable lump present arises, in around 5 per cent of cases, from a very small breast cancer in the *in situ* phase (*see* Chapter 2);

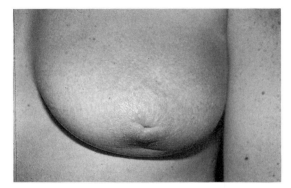

Figure 3.2 Skin tether from an underlying carcinoma

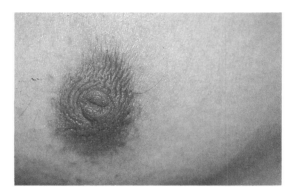

Figure 3.3 Retraction of nipple, benign cause

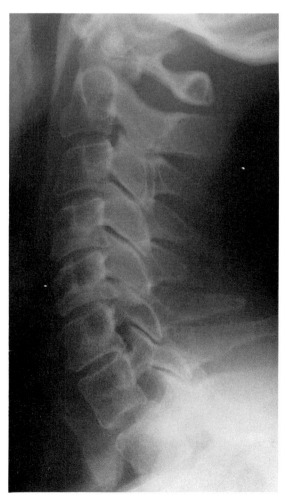

Figure 3.1 Cervical spondylitis: narrowing of C4/5 and C5/6 disc spaces and posterior osteophyte formation

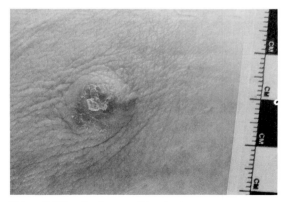

Figure 3.4 Paget's disease of the nipple

more commonly it is caused by duct ectasia (*see* Chapters 2, 6 and 8) or by duct papillomas (*see* Chapter 2). The discharge may be milky, clear yellow, thick and green, purulent or fresh blood – the type of discharge is not helpful in diagnosis.

The nipple may become eczematous with a red, raw appearance. This is caused by Paget's disease of the nipple (*see* Chapter 2) which denotes carcinoma in the underlying ducts (*Figure 3.4*). The other cause of nipple soreness is when a woman with an indrawn nipple does not properly clean it (which is done both by flattening the nipple and using 'baby buds').

Examination of the breast

Examination of the breast is first by observation.

The woman sits on the edge of the examination couch facing the examiner (or if she is self-examining she stands facing a full length mirror). The breasts are inspected for: a lump; skin tether; indrawing of the nipple; inflammation; nipple eczema.

The woman then raises her arms slowly away from the body until they are above her head; during this the breasts are inspected for any skin tether or the heightening of a lump. If no abnormality is seen but the complaint is of a lump, the examiner should ask the patient where she feels the lump and then to repeat the procedure with careful observation of the area indicated.

A woman complaining of a nipple discharge is asked to squeeze the breast to produce the discharge. The examiner may then press each point around the areola to try to locate where the discharge is coming from.

To palpate the breasts one of us (JC) prefers to start with the patient lying on the couch flat, another (RWB) prefers to prop the patient up with pillows to around 35 degrees. For breast self-examination (BSE) we suggest that a woman rests on two pillows. Examination is made with the flat of the fingers, not by digging in the tips nor by picking up breast tissue between the fingers. The examiner begins with the breast opposite to that complained of; the breast is examined in all four quadrants plus the axillary tail and the nipple area. Again we differ slightly: one of us prefers to feel each area by downward pressure, the other to use circular rotation of the fingers while examining. We suggest the latter to women for self-examination – working in along each hour of the clock hand towards the nipple. If the examiner is in doubt the examination is repeated with the woman's hands above her head.

Finally, the woman is asked to sit up and lean slightly forwards and the breasts are re-examined. This is particularly useful in distinguishing a true lump from lumpy tissue; a true lump can be felt from underneath – 'weighed' in the hand.

If the examiner cannot feel a lump then the patient is asked to 'put one finger on the lump'. When she is sure she can feel it the examiner places his finger exactly where indicated. Here lies a useful tip: if a woman asked to put one finger on the lump immediately does so, then she probably has a genuine lump. If she feels around – often with several fingers – and says 'it's somewhere here' then she probably has not.

It is important to make a decision as to whether a definite lump is present or not before any further investigative procedures are carried out such as needle biopsy. It is useful to realize that the decision that a true lump is present will ultimately mean that it has to be removed (unless it is a cyst and is drained).

The categories after examination are:

1. A lump is present or has a sign that needs further investigation, e.g. skin tether.
2. The breast is normal.
3. The breast is generally lumpy; while no definite lump can be felt it is difficult to exclude or the breast has a lumpy area (indefinite edges, not certainly a lump but prominent) where the patient indicates. This category should be kept as small as possible: the examiner must try to be definite about the other categories.

Then, the lines of procedure are:

1. *A lump is present* – needling to see if cystic; then, if solid, there must be a tissue diagnosis (cytology or Trucut needle biopsy, *see below*) and a mammogram is taken.
2. *Normal* – woman reassured and discharged.
3. *Lumpy* – re-examine the breast at a different time of the menstrual cycle (2 weeks later) and take a mammogram.

A competent and confident examiner should be able to place around 80 per cent of the cases in the first two categories. In our programme of self-referral after BSE the radiographer examines and decides between normal (patient discharged after a mammogram) and abnormal. Both abnormal categories (definitely abnormality and lumpy breast) are seen by the clinic doctor, although in the case of a definite abnormality a radiographer experienced in clinical examination could certainly carry on to diagnostic procedures such as cytology.

Without further investigation a good idea of the final diagnosis can be formed after clinical examination in the symptomatic referral clinic. Age and menopausal status are important in this: cysts do not occur after the menopause. The likely diagnoses of a genuine lump are:

1. Young woman – from the menarche to around 30 – with a smooth, very mobile, often ellipsoid, breast lump ranging in size from 0.5 to 3 cm in diameter = **fibroadenoma** (*Figure 3.5*).
2. Woman after menopause = **carcinoma**.
3. Woman from 35 to 50 = **cyst** (or) **carcinoma.**

A cyst typically will feel smooth, rounded and relatively mobile. The fluid is too tense to give clinical signs of fluid and the lump will feel like a solid lump. The cyst may feel irregular when it is surrounded by dysplastic tissue and the way to both investigate and confirm that a breast lump is cystic is to needle it (*see* Chapter 13).

Most carcinomas present as a solid lump and a minority show the classic features of skin or deep tether or nipple indrawing. However when there is such fixity then the lump is almost certainly a carcinoma.

The breast may show the signs of a locally advanced carcinoma with skin oedema (*peau d'orange* – orange skin appearance with the sweat gland pores prominent, *Figure 3.6*) or skin ulceration (*Figure 3.7*). Such a growth may be fixed to the chest wall or to the pectoralis muscle – shown by asking the woman to place her hand on her hip and press.

Examination of the axillary lymph nodes has not been described because this is a prognostic rather than a diagnostic manoeuvre. The decision as to whether there is a lesion in the breast or not relies on examination of the breast itself! If the axillary nodes have carcinoma in them, then the prognosis of a breast cancer is worse (*see* Chapter 1). To examine the axillary nodes, the hand is placed flat in the axilla with the fingers reaching as high as possible, the right hand to left axilla and vice versa. The patient is encouraged to relax and her hand is placed by her side to prevent the axillary skin being tensed. The hand is then swept down the axilla while the fingers push. An alternative is to sit the patient up, approach from behind and put a hand in each axilla.

Examination of the breast may be by slightly differing techniques, but the principles are uniform. The only way to become competent is to carry out frequent examinations and to see the variety of clinical signs. The radiographers in our Helen Garrod Unit attended the referral clinic and ward rounds of patients about to be operated on for several months before they began lecturing on BSE and began making clinical decisions on women self-referring.

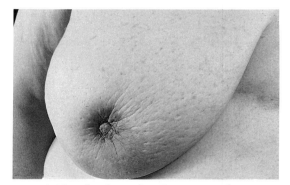

Figure 3.6 Locally advanced carcinoma: *peau d'orange*

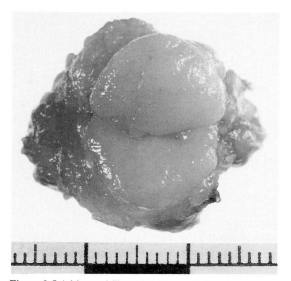

Figure 3.5 A bisected fibroadenoma: note the sharp, smooth edge and white, bulging, homogeneous cut surface

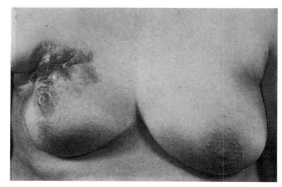

Figure 3.7 Locally advanced carcinoma: ulceration

4

The diagnosis of breast cancer

As discussed in Chapter 3, breast cancer may present in a variety of ways: as a lump, a mammographic abnormality, soreness of the nipple, discharge from the nipple and as metastasis in distant sites or in axillary nodes. By far the commonest of these is a breast lump. Mammographic abnormalities leading to the diagnosis of cancer are increasing as screening programmes are introduced. Soreness of the nipple due to underlying Paget's disease accounts for only 1 per cent of the breast cancer in Nottingham. Discharge from the nipple has led to only twelve cancers being diagnosed (out of approximately 3000); distant metastasis with a previously unrecognized small palpable primary has been seen only three times as the presenting sign. Metastasis to axillary nodes without palpable lump has accounted for nine presentations.

Breast lump

Unfortunately, in the enthusiasm for newer methods of diagnosis, patients complaining of breast lumps are often improperly managed. Again referring to Chapter 3, the first decision that the clinician must make is whether a lump is present or not. Under no circumstances should the clinician decide that a lump 'may' be present, proceed to needling and then decide (because no fluid is aspirated) that no lump is present after all.

This point has been restated and stressed because we feel strongly that it is an important principle. Clear thinking and definite decisions must be made and there must be no abdication from clinical decision by substitution of mammography.

Once the decision is made that a lump is present then the surgeon proceeds on a set path. A 21-gauge needle is advanced into the lump and an attempt is made to aspirate fluid; if a lump proves to be a cyst and disappears completely on aspiration (and this is usually the case) then no further action is taken and the woman is reassured. If the lump has not disappeared completely then investigation is required: usually to re-examine after 1 week. If the lump is solid on needling, the surgeon proceeds to Trucut needle biopsy or to fine needle aspiration cytology (FNAC).

Trucut needle biopsy

Trucut biopsy is carried out under local anaesthetic with adrenaline 1 in 100 000. A skin bleb is raised and local anaesthetic is also injected into the lump. A small incision is made through the bleb with the tip of a sharp scalpel blade. The Trucut needle is pushed, closed, through the skin incision and a biopsy of the lump is taken as in *Figure 4.1*. Following biopsy the patient is instructed to apply firm pressure for 10 minutes – this prevents bruising. Fortunately a carcinoma is easier to biopsy than a benign lump – the carcinoma being hard and cutting easily, while benign tissue has the consistency of firm indiarubber; fibroadenomas are often too firm to push the needle into at all. *Figure 4.2* shows a typical specimen obtained from a carcinoma. The core is suitable for histological examination, which can be carried out in any district general hospital.

With the exception of abscess and tissue showing the changes of pregnancy, and in certain cases of fibroadenoma (*see* Chapter 13), a report of benign

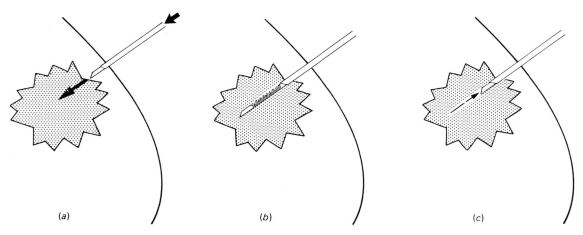

(a)   (b)   (c)

Figure 4.1 The procedure of Trucut biopsy of a breast lump: a small skin incision is made and the whole needle tip advanced as far as the lump (*a*). The central needle is then pushed through the lump (*b*), a piece of tissue falling into the slot. The outer sheath is then advanced over this and the closed needle withdrawn (*c*)

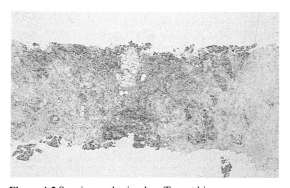

Figure 4.2 Specimen obtained on Trucut biopsy

tissue, or a report of an unsatisfactory core for examination, is followed by excision of the lump. A report of invasive carcinoma is followed without further diagnostic procedure by the appropriate treatment.

Trucut biopsy has overall proved very accurate (*Table 4.1*). In three-quarters of the patients with cancerous breast lumps a definite preoperative

Table 4.1 Reports on Trucut biopsies in 932 cases subsequently confirmed as cancer

Trucut diagnosis	No. of cases	Percentage
Carcinoma	708	76
Suspicious	44	5
Benign	180	19
Total	932	100

diagnosis has been obtained. An advantage is that frozen-section examination of lumps at operation has largely been dropped in our unit and is only used in cases where there is a high index of suspicion. We are particularly pleased to have rid ourselves of frozen-section examinations; we find it unacceptable to carry out routine frozen section for breast lumps, causing unnecessary anxiety to many patients who ultimately are proved to have benign lumps. A preoperative diagnosis of cancer allows a full discussion with the patient and her husband and they may participate in decisions regarding the form of primary treatment.

Trucut biopsy is not satisfactory for all lesions. Small or hard rubbery lumps give unsatisfactory cores – the needle being deflected off the lump itself.

Fine needle aspiration cytology

A preoperative diagnosis may also be achieved using fine needle aspiration cytology (FNAC). A variety of techniques has been described, but that most frequently used is as follows: a 21-gauge 40-mm needle is attached to a 10-ml syringe and introduced into the lump through the skin without local anaesthetic. Suction is applied and the needle is passed into the lump in several directions. Suction is released and the needle withdrawn from the breast. The syringe is detached and the contents expelled onto a microscope slide and a smear made in a similar way to that used for a blood film. Smears are air dried and stained (*Figures 4.3* and *4.4*).

The problem of this technique lies in the interpretation. A pathologist who has taken the time to become expert at reading breast cytology is required and not every hospital will have one. Training in reading cervical cytology cannot be simply translated to reading breast cytology. Cytology gives the diagnosis in over 90 per cent of palpable breast cancers; however, very occasionally benign lumps are falsely diagnosed as cancer.

We act on a cytological diagnosis of cancer when this is compatible with the clinical and/or mammographic appearance. However, if the lump might be a fibroadenoma clinically (*see* Chapter 3), then we always have the safeguard of a full histological diagnosis.

We also occasionally use cytology to avoid removing benign lesions (such as clinically obvious fibroadenomas in young women). In doing this, a very clear protocol has to be drawn in order not to miss the occasional carcinoma clinically resembling a fibroadenoma. The protocol is described fully in Chapter 13.

Diagnosis from mammography

We have already emphasized the point that mammography is not a diagnostic method for use in the referral clinic. Mammography in this instance may occasionally prove a useful adjunct, but should never be used to over-ride clear clinical decisions. Mammography is, however, the basis of breast-screening programmes. It is a very efficient method of detecting impalpable carcinomas (*Figure 4.5; see* Chapter 10). Such lesions shown only on mammography are removed by 'marker biopsy'. The radiographer places superior and lateral skin markers over the estimated levels of the abnormality and takes mediolateral and craniocaudal check

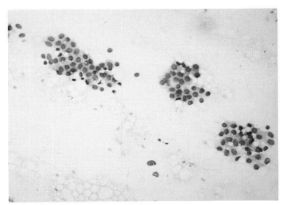

Figure 4.3 Benign cells from fine needle aspiration. The cells form cohesive clumps and nuclei are regular. Occasional 'bare' nuclei are present. May–Grunwald–Giesma, ×156

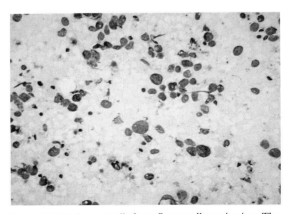

Figure 4.4 Malignant cells from fine needle aspiration. The cells are dispersed, with marked nuclear pleomorphism. May–Grunwald–Giesma, ×156

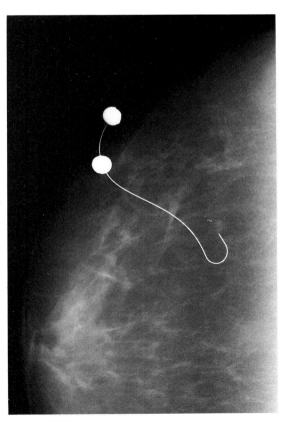

Figure 4.5 Mammogram of an impalpable cancer marked under mammographic control

X-rays. The radiologist then places a needle through the estimated position of the abnormality; further check X-rays are taken and the needle readjusted if necessary. The direction of the needle should be parallel to the chest wall and not directed towards the chest.

A number of different needles may be used for this procedure. Currently we are using the Frank needle (Wm Cook, Denmark). This is a hooked wire inside a needle for introduction. The hook engages the wire in the tissues so that it cannot be inadvertently pulled out.

An alternative we have recently introduced – which is easier for the unpractised radiologist and which also makes surgery easier – is to place markers over the abnormality in the craniocaudal and mediolateral planes, and then to place two spinal needles and check their position. Ideally, they should cross just behind the lesion. At operation the assistant holds the needles firmly and the surgeon cuts down onto them.

In order to keep the ratio of benign to malignant biopsies to a reasonable level, the radiologist should grade his reporting and not simply (as is often done) report the presence of any abnormality (*see* Chapter 6). In our centre, if EJR grades the mammograms as 'definite' or 'probable malignancy' and there is no palpable lump, then marker biopsy is carried out. If the report is 'indeterminate', where the likelihood of the lesion being malignant is around 40 to 1, then we carry out mammographic follow-up over a 6-month period.

In 4 years (1982–85), 94 marker biopsies have been carried out in our unit, resulting in the diagnosis of 24 carcinomas.

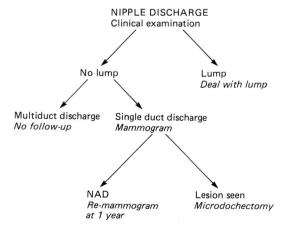

Figure 4.6 Management of nipple discharge

Paget's disease of the nipple

Paget's disease of the nipple (*see* Chapters 2 and 3) should be suspected in any patient with a raw appearance of the nipple – sometimes restricted to the nipple and sometimes extending to the areola. Some of these cases have a palpable lump, which is investigated as above. The remainder are investigated by nipple biopsy, which is simply taken in the referral clinic with a sharp scalpel blade under local anaesthetic containing a little adrenaline to diminish skin bleeding.

Nipple discharge

Few carcinomas present as nipple discharge alone, although it is a symptom often stressed in women's magazines. In fact, in the Nottingham clinic only 12 carcinomas have been discovered from investigation of nipple discharge alone. A patient complaining of nipple discharge is first examined. If a lump is found then the case becomes an investigation of that lump, as previously described. If no lump is found, then a mammogram is taken.

The line of management we have then adopted is first to separate discharge from physiological disorder from discharge of pathological abnormality (*Figure 4.6*). A bilateral or multiduct discharge has been classified as the former and, apart from being kept under observation, has not received any special investigation.

A single-duct discharge, on the other hand, is further investigated. If the mammogram is clear a further mammogram is taken 1 year later. If the mammogram shows an abnormality then we carry out microdochectomy. This procedure may be carried out under local anaesthetic. The discharging duct is freed at the nipple and a suture placed at the skin end and tied tightly around the probe. A radial incision is then made along the probe across the nipple and areola and continued outside the areola. The duct is dissected free of the breast fat with blunt scissors and followed as far as possible. The duct is then opened with a small pair of sharp scissors.

We have reviewed 170 cases of single duct discharge in all of which we carried out microdochectomy (*Table 4.2*). Twelve cancers were diagnosed and all were at a very favourable stage (intraduct carcinoma only with no invasion). Ten of the twelve had preoperative mammograms and on eight of these the carcinoma showed as a mammographic abnormality. It is for this reason that we have altered our policy for treatment to operation only when the mammogram is abnormal and to otherwise perform follow-up mammography. If we had followed this policy we would have had 30 in place of 170 microdochectomies to carry out.

The causes of single duct discharge are shown in *Table 4.2*.

Table 4.2 The final diagnosis in 170 cases of single duct nipple discharge without palpable lump

Number of patients	Pathological diagnosis
12	Ductal carcinoma *in situ*
73	Intraduct papilloma
73	Benign breast disease
12	Normal breast tissue

Breast cancer presenting as metastasis

Approximately 3000 breast cancers have come under our care in the last 13 years. Nine have presented as enlarged axillary nodes showing adenocarcinoma on histological examination, but with no palpable breast mass. Mammography showed an abnormality in some of these. All proved to have cancers in the ipsilateral breast.

Three cases were diagnosed after presenting initially as distant metastases without an obvious breast lump, but in all a small, although in fact palpable, primary breast cancer was present.

5

Mammographic equipment and technique

Equipment for X-ray mammography

X-ray mammography is the accepted method of imaging the breast in symptomatic women. It can demonstrate occult disease and is considered the choice for breast screening. To produce mammograms of the highest quality, the radiographer should be properly trained and the equipment used should be appropriate for the mammographic examination. Poor positioning, compression or the use of inappropriate image receptors or X-ray tubes will result in an inadequate image. Contrast and resolution are important features of the image because of the subtle changes in tissue absorption and, in particular, to visualize microcalcifications indicative of early malignant disease.

In mammography, the radiation dose must be as low as possible. The breast is imaged using low photon energies for high contrast; however, high photon energies are needed to reduce dose. Careful selection of X-ray equipment, filters and receptors will reach a compromise where contrast and resolution are optimum with a low radiation dose. Frequent quality control and dose measurements must be carried out (*see* Chapter 7).

The X-ray machine

There are many different manufacturers producing dedicated mammography machines (*Figure 5.1*) and each unit has to choose according to their individual requirements. The choice will depend on whether screening or examination of symptomatic women is to be carried out. Screening covers large numbers of asymptomatic women and images need to be taken

quickly and easily. The handling characteristics of commercially available units vary in the ease of use. The need to reach a population to be screened is important so that mobile cabins and vans are used in some screening programmes. In symptomatic mammography, the need is for more sophisticated

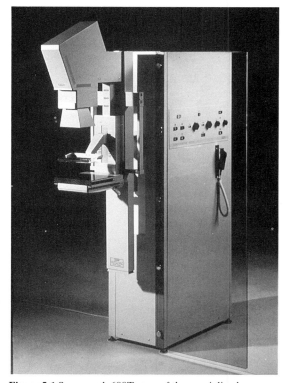

Figure 5.1 Senograph 600T: one of the specialized machines for mammography (reproduced courtesy of IGE Medical Systems Ltd)

equipment with a magnification facility. There are special 'add on' facilities for some mammography machines for stereotactic localization of impalpable lesions for fine needle aspiration cytology or accurate marking by a special hooked wire for excision biopsy. In these centres ultrasound and Lite-scanning machines may be present as complementary techniques.

The steady improvement in the quality of the mammographic image in recent years has been due to advances in film/screen technology and refinement of the mammographic unit.

A dedicated unit is required to provide the X-ray spectrum necessary. The choice of spectrum depends on the receptor. For film/screen combinations, an X-ray tube with molybdenum target and molybdenum filter is conventionally used. For xeromammography, a tungsten anode with an aluminium filter is used. Molybdenum has characteristic X-rays at 17.4 and 19.4 keV and a K edge at 20 keV; there is a large increase in the photoelectronic absorption in the filter at its K edge and a

corresponding decrease in transmission and the X-ray spectrum is therefore much attenuated above 20 keV (*Figure 5.2*). A peak kilovoltage in the range 26–30 kV is usually employed. The molybdenum target/molybdenum filter tube is well suited to small or medium breasts. Larger breasts require a higher energy spectrum because they absorb most of the low energy photons, increasing the required dose and lowering the contrast. This spectrum can be achieved by using a palladium filter (K edge 24.3 keV) which is used with either molybdenum or tungsten target (*Figure 5.3*); its spectrum gives slightly less contrast than the molybdenum/molybdenum combination, with a reduction in dose. Dose reductions of up to 50 per cent have been reported for tungsten target/palladium filter combination and 35 per cent dose reduction for molybdenum target/palladium filter. However, the unit with molybdenum target/molybdenum filter has a higher contrast when imaging the normal-sized breast.

The overall unsharpness of the image will depend on the unsharpness of the receptor, the size of the focal spot of the X-ray tube and patient movement. Patient movement is minimized by good compression. The geometric unsharpness should match, or be better than, the receptor unsharpness and a focal spot size of less than 0.5 mm, with a focus/film

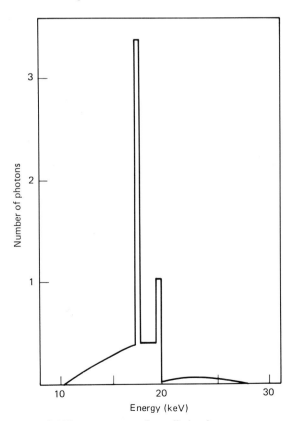

Figure 5.2 Photon spectrum for radiation from a molybdenum target at 28 kV. Filtered by 30-μm molybdenum

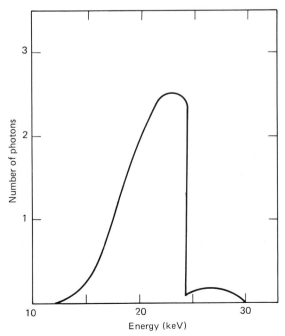

Figure 5.3 Photon spectrum for radiation from a tungsten target at 30 kV filtered by 50-μm palladium

distance of 60 cm, is required. For magnification, a focal spot size of 0.1 mm is now commonplace.

Since mammographic equipment is constantly evolving, covers a wide price range and may be required for differing situations, it is unwise to make specific recommendations. In starting a unit the work to be undertaken has first to be considered. The radiographer and radiologist should then assess the available machines. There are several machines on the market ranging from £23 000 for a basic machine to £50 000 for one with magnification and grid. After the choice of machine, the most suitable receptor is then decided.

Magnification mammography

In magnification mammography an air gap is introduced between breast and receptor to produce a magnified image (*Figure 5.4*). This technique is proving increasingly useful in the differentiation between benign and malignant disease. The nature of microcalcification particles can be better assessed (*Figure 5.5*), small changes in architectural distortion analysed by disassociating the various planes of breast tissue and the demonstration of multifocal disease or possible adjacent intraduct disease (which have a bearing on the surgical management of patients) are important uses of this technique. It is essential to have a small focal spot size, 0.1 mm, and a magnification of ×2 is recommended; with this combination the effective unsharpness would be improved by approximately 35 per cent. Using suitable filtration, e.g. palladium, of the primary beam helps to compensate for the increase in dose, bringing it to an acceptable level.

Receptors

Screens/films

Mammographic imaging systems should be able to image microcalcifications smaller than 200 µm and specially designed screens are used. A single screen is used to avoid cross-over and is placed behind the film. More photons interact in the front half of the screen than in the back half and this configuration brings the production point of the fluorescent light photons as close as possible to the emulsion. There is a trend to faster screen/film combinations with an increase in contrast without loss of definition resulting in a lower dose. Good contact between screen and film is essential. Current cassette materials and design help to decrease the radiation dose. Screens are available with rare earth phosphors, e.g. Kodak Min. R, and these can be fitted

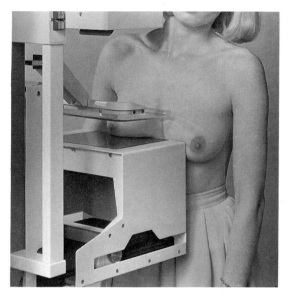

Figure 5.4 Magnification technique: an air gap is introduced between object and film to give a macro-image

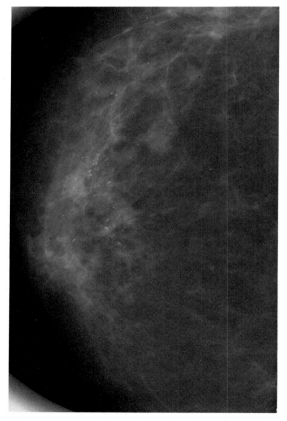

Figure 5.5 Magnification view showing microcalcification indicative of malignancy

into specially designed mammography cassettes which allow optimum film/screen contact. Vacuum packaging in light, tight, plastic bags can also be used. Screens need to be kept scrupulously clean or else artefacts will be produced on the film.

The sensitivity of the screen is determined by the X-ray absorption characteristics and light production efficiency, and depends on the efficiency with which the energy absorbed is converted to light. The wavelength spectrum of the fluorescent light photons emitted by the screen depends on the phosphor used. For maximum sensitivity the spectral response of the film should be matched to the light emitted by the screening.

The films used with radiographic screens are predominantly blue sensitive. Screen films are suitable for automatic development usually at 90 seconds and can be processed under normal darkroom safe light conditions. It is recommended that a dedicated processor is used for processing mammography film.

Xeroradiography

Xeroradiography (*Figure 5.6*) is also used as a receptor in mammography. This is a dry non-silver process which uses a higher energy spectrum from a tungsten target; 40–50 kV is used with additional filtration of aluminium. The image receptor is a plate of selenium which is uniformly precharged and sealed in a light, tight cassette in a special machine (the conditioner). A latent image is formed by photoconductive discharge as the plate is placed under the breast and exposed to radiation. The charge pattern is developed in a second machine (the processor) by dusting with blue powder or

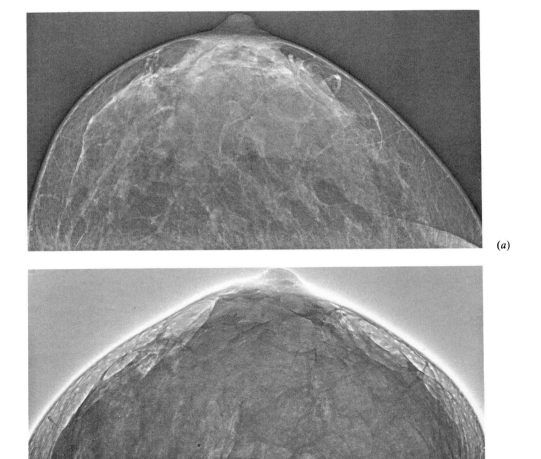

(a)

(b)

Figure 5.6 Xeromammogram showing microcalcification. (*a*) Negative mode; (*b*) positive mode

liquid (toner); the toner particles are charged by friction and are attracted by the charge on the surface of the selenium. A positive or a negative image may be produced. In positive mode, the more highly charged areas corresponding to the denser parts of the breast are dark blue (*Figure 5.6b*), in negative mode the denser areas are lighter blue (*Figure 5.6a*). The image is transferred from the selenium plate to paper by contact and sealed for viewing. There is a reduction in dose, when using negative mode, of about 30 per cent.

Xerographs (*Figure 5.6b*) show less contrast between large areas of different density, but show marked enhancement in the vicinity of any sharp changes in contrast. This is known as edge enhancement which can assist in the visualization of microcalcifications and differences in tissue absorption.

Mammographic grids

The contrast and film definition are reduced because of scattered radiation. Specially designed mammographic grids can significantly reduce the scatter so that contrast and definition improve. Both stationary and moving grids are available. The use of these

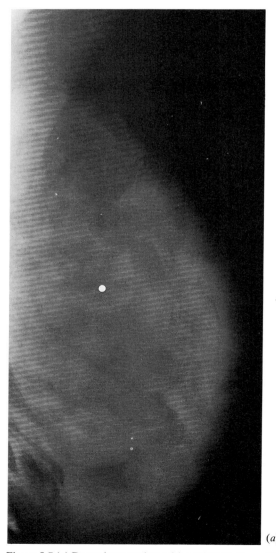

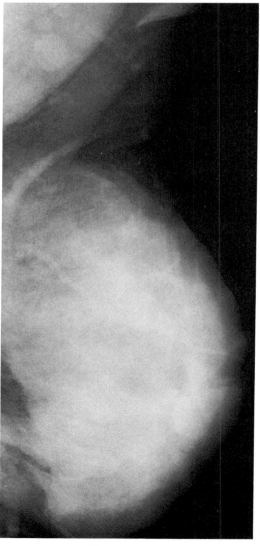

(a)

(b)

Figure 5.7 (*a*) Dense breast taken with a grid technique; (*b*) same breast without a grid

increases the dose by up to 2.5 times. Palladium filters will help to reduce this and keep it within accepted limits. The improvement in the image is very important particularly in the dense breast (*Figures 5.7a, b*).

Technique

X-ray mammography is not a difficult technique; however, careful positioning and some dedication is needed to provide mammograms where the whole breast is imaged with optimum detail for subtle changes to be recognized. It is recommended that a room be dedicated for mammography; this should be light, airy and as pleasant as possible. The equipment is purpose built and specially trained radiographers are needed to operate it. The radiographer is an important member of the team in the diagnosis of breast disease and close cooperation with the radiologist, surgeon and pathologist is desirable.

A mammogram can be uncomfortable and even painful. The procedure should be carried out as efficiently and quickly as possible to minimize the discomfort. The patients need compassionate but firm handling and, to obtain full cooperation, the radiographer should be friendly and explain fully what is required and what to expect.

Films with high contrast and wide tonal range to show the skin and deeper structures of the breast on the one image are necessary.

The breast varies in size and composition. It may be composed of predominantly fatty or glandular tissue – on the image these vary considerably according to compression. Compression of the breast is sometimes unpleasant for the patient; however, firm compression is important for the reduction of dose, contrast is improved because the scattered radiation is reduced, the unsharpness of the image is improved because the breast is closer to the receptor and there is a reduction in the range of densities in the image. Adequate compression is therefore very important and even, firm pressure, without excessive discomfort to the patient, should be the aim of the radiographer.

Correct annotations and the patient's name, date of birth and date of X-ray should be clearly seen on all radiographs.

There are two categories of patients for mammography:

1. Asymptomatic screening women – these are well women who have to be X-rayed quickly, efficiently with a high through-put achieved in the interest of economy.
2. Symptomatic patients or patients with a previous history of breast pathology – these patients require a much more sympathetic approach since more are anxious and some are obviously distressed.

For screening the asymptomatic woman the erect 45 degree lateral oblique is the view usually adopted.

The technique for 45 degree lateral oblique

The machine is angled to 45 degrees from the horizontal position (*Figure 5.8*). Sometimes patients with small breasts can be positioned more accurately with the tube angled to 30–35 degrees. The patient stands facing the machine with the edge of the film against the lateral chest wall and the arm nearest the machine resting on a convenient part of the equipment with the elbow bent. The patient is leaned towards the film, the top edge of the film is into the axilla and the lower edge one inch below the inframammary fold. The breast is firmly lifted and the patient's position adjusted until the lateral side of the breast is resting against the film with the nipple in profile. Any overlapping abdominal skin or fat encroaching into the image area should be removed at this stage. The breast is pushed firmly up and forward away from the chest wall with the flat hand and compression should be applied until the breast tissue is of even thickness. In women with large breasts, it may be necessary to use more than one film to completely image the whole breast.

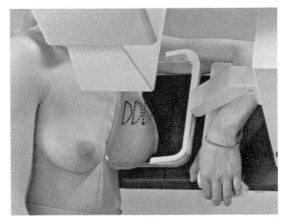

Figure 5.8 Patient positioned for 45° mediolateral oblique. This view provides a good demonstration of mammary lesions, rib cage area and axillary space

The correctly positioned radiograph (*Figure 5.9*) will show all the breast tissue from the axillary to the inframammary fold with the pectoral muscle visible at the base of the breast to nipple level and the nipple in profile with skin detail.

This view with its high sensitivity, the ability to produce the maximum amount of information on a single film with low patient dose and the ability to easily reproduce the image, makes it ideal and economical for screening.

To take an X-ray of the symptomatic patient, a two-view technique is generally used. In our centre the 45 degree lateral oblique view is performed together with a craniocaudal (CC) view. In some centres the oblique view is replaced by the erect mediolateral view. This view is combined with the CC view for marker biopsy.

The technique for the craniocaudal view

The patient stands or sits facing the X-ray machine and is rotated 15–20 degrees towards the cassette (*Figure 5.10*). The patient's arm on the side to be examined is extended and flexed with the shoulder relaxed and the hand resting on a suitable part of the machine. The breast is lifted and the patient brought forward, the machine is raised until the edge of the cassette is placed in the inframammary fold and the breast is rested on top of the cassette with the nipple in profile (in some patients this may not be possible in which case the whole breast is imaged and profile views of the nipple and retroareola area are taken separately). While the radiographer is adjusting the position, the patient is asked to lean forward so that the whole breast is gradually placed on to the film. Compression is applied until the breast is firmly held with an even thickness throughout.

The correctly positioned radiograph will show the maximum amount of tissue with the nipple in profile (*Figure 5.11*).

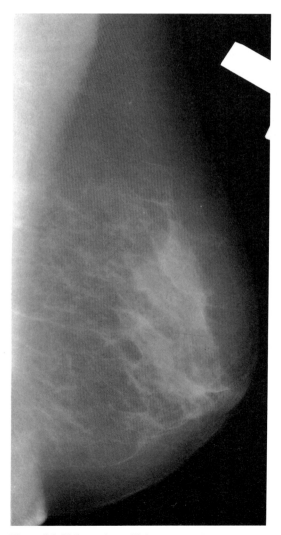

Figure 5.9 Oblique view will show pectoral muscle to nipple level; nipple in profile; axillary tail of breast; inframammary fold

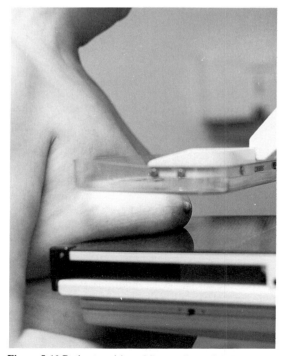

Figure 5.10 Patient positioned for craniocaudal view

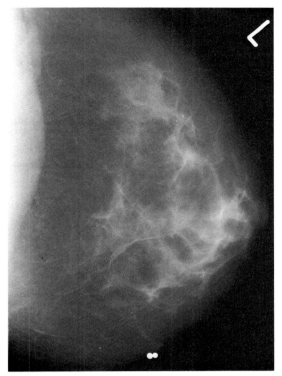

Figure 5.11 Craniocaudal view will show nipple in profile; breast tissue medial to lateral aspect; small amount of chest wall fat

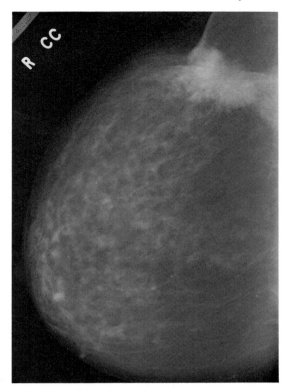

Figure 5.12 Extended craniocaudal: more lateral breast tissue and axillary tail

The extended craniocaudal view (lateral extension)

To view abnormalities in the lateral aspect of the breast, the patient is positioned initially for the craniocaudal view and is then rotated approximately 60 degrees away from the cassette so that only the lateral aspect of the breast is against the front edge of the machine. The breast is lifted and the patient brought forward until the chest wall is in contact with the cassette. The breast is placed onto the cassette with the nipple in profile. Compression is applied while easing the axilla into the field with the patient's arm and shoulder relaxed. The medial part of the breast may not be seen on this image (*Figure 5.12*).

Technique for the erect mediolateral view (as a true lateral projection)

This view (the ML view) can be used for localization procedures (prior to biopsy).

The machine is set into the vertical position. The patient sits or stands facing the equipment and is rotated 45 degrees away from the machine with the arm of the side to be examined resting on a convenient part of the machine (*Figure 5.13*). The lower edge of the cassette is 2 inches (5.3 cm) below the inframammary fold. The breast is lifted, pulled forward, up and away from the chest wall, with the patient leaning forward and gently rotating until the lateral aspect of the breast is resting against the cassette. Compression is applied while holding the breast with a flat hand, withdrawing this as the compression holds the breast firmly and gives an even thickness throughout. The correctly positioned radiograph shows inframammary fold, pectoral muscle and nipple in profile (*Figure 5.14*).

Technique for lateromedial view

This view (the LM view) can be used as an alternative to the mediolateral and is used to demonstrate lesions in the medial aspect of the breast. The machine is set to the vertical position with the patient standing or sitting facing the machine. The arm of the side to be examined is

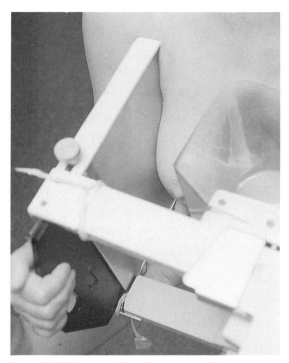

Figure 5.13 Patient positioned for erect mediolateral view

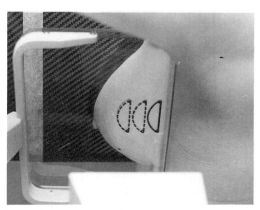

Figure 5.15 Patient positioned for the lateromedial view

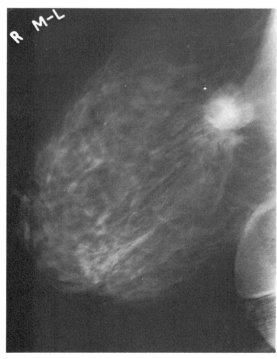

Figure 5.14 Mediolateral view will show nipple in profile; pectoral muscle; inframammary fold

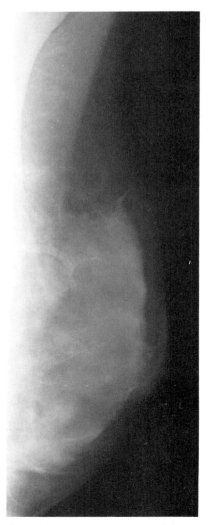

Figure 5.16 Lateromedial view will show nipple in profile; pectoral muscle; inframammary fold

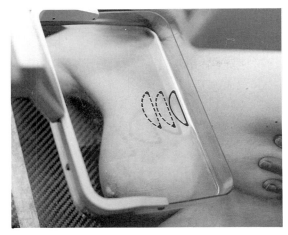

Figure 5.17 Patient positioned for axillary view

raised and placed on a convenient part of the machine. The cassette is placed between the patient's breasts (*Figure 5.15*). The lower edge of the cassette is 1–2 inches (2.6–5.2 cm) below the inframammary fold. The breast is lifted and pulled forward away from the chest wall, and the patient is rotated until the medial part of the breast is resting against the cassette with the nipple in profile. The breast is supported with the flat hand and compression is firmly applied withdrawing the hand as the compression holds the breast and produces an even thickness throughout.

The correctly positioned image will show all the breast tissue with the pectoral muscle; however, it is more difficult to position the nipple in profile in this view (*Figure 5.16*).

Technique for the axillary tail oblique view

The equipment is set as for the 45 degree lateral oblique. The patient is similarly positioned (*Figure 5.17*), but is not rotated as far towards the machine which is placed higher than for the normal oblique view. Compression is applied with the shoulder relaxed.

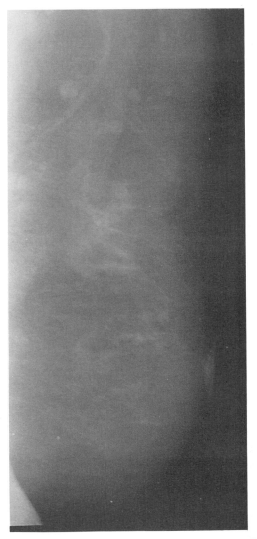

Figure 5.18 Axillary view will show low axilla and axillary tail

The correctly positioned radiograph will show the axillary tail of the breast and most of the axilla (*Figure 5.18*).

6

Mammography – reading and interpretation

There is a wealth of information recorded on a mammogram, and to read and interpret the displayed information accurately requires both meticulous attention to detail and experience.

It is important to know what questions are being asked, so that answers can be provided without also giving a mass of confusing information.

The most common questions are:

1. What is the cause of this woman's symptoms? Lumpiness, pain and discharge are the most frequently encountered symptoms.
2. Is a lesion detected by the clinician solitary or multifocal or an area of a diffuse process? The actual nature of a lesion itself is quite likely to be resolved by other methods, Trucut biopsy or aspiration cytology for instance, but it is most important to know if it is localized or if others are present.
3. Is there any abnormality present in this asymptomatic woman's breast?

It is worth while reiterating an important maxim: whatever question is asked must be answered.

There may be information judged to be relevant in addition to that specifically requested, which is worth imparting to the initiator of the request for a mammogram. Above all a clear unequivocal opinion must be given whenever possible. It may, in some instances, be necessary to advise further management, such as a repeat mammogram after an interval or an ultrasound examination.

Whatever question is asked the actual process of viewing the mammogram is the same. It is a two-stage process: first, film reading to detect an abnormality and then interpretation of the abnormalities detected.

Film reading

To undertake film reading accurately, it is necessary to progress through several well-defined steps.

Step 1

Check the film quality. Is all the breast tissue demonstrated or should, for example, an extended craniocaudal view be taken in order to demonstrate the lateral half of the breasts (*Figure 6.1a, b*).

Step 2

Check the patient's name and age. A rounded lesion in a 35-year-old is likely to be a fibroadenoma, but in a 65-year-old the identical appearance should be interpreted as a probable carcinoma (*Figure 6.2a, b*).

Step 3

Determine the normal mammographic background pattern for the patient:

- Is involution complete or partial?
- Is there cystic dysplasia present in both breasts?

These observations will influence interpretation (*Figure 6.3a, b, c*).

Step 4

Check the breasts for symmetry (beware previous surgery which will result in a reduction of breast tissue). Particularly important is asymmetry of the duct shadow, but also note the shape of the glandular tissue and any asymmetry of density.

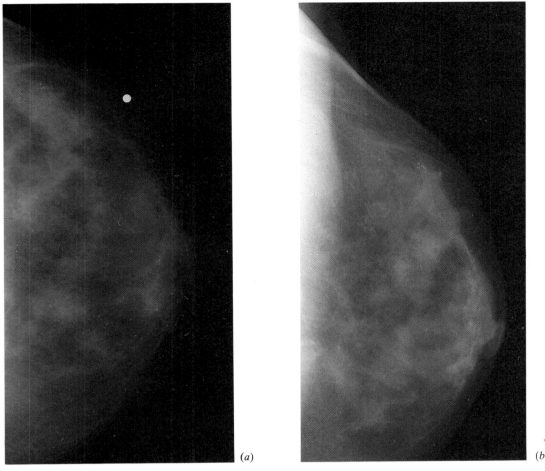

(a)

(b)

Figure 6.1 (*a*) Craniocaudal view showing microcalcification in lateral breast. (*b*) Extended craniocaudal view showing more axillary tail and better demonstration of the microcalcification

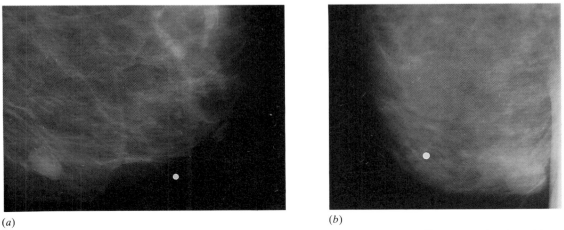

(a)

(b)

Figure 6.2 (*a*) 35-year-old patient with rounded lesion which proved to be a fibroadenoma; (*b*) 57-year-old patient with rounded density which proved to be a mucoid carcinoma

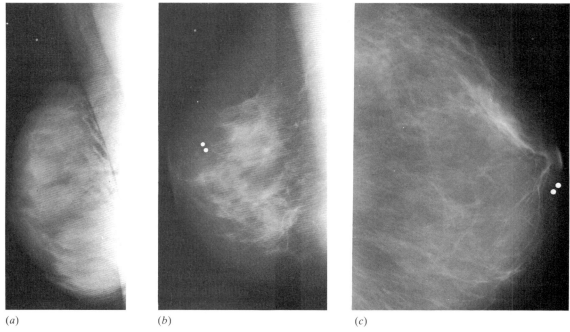

(a)   (b)   (c)

Figure 6.3 (*a*) Very little involution of glandular tissue;
(*b*) partial involution of glandular tissue; (*c*) total involution of glandular tissue

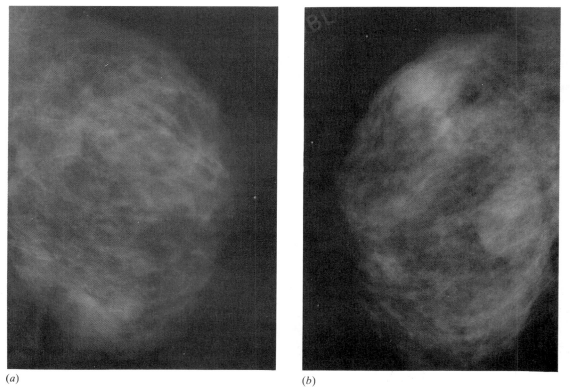

(a)   (b)

Figure 6.4 Showing asymmetrical densities in (*a*) left and (*b*) right breasts

By this stage, it is probable that any lesion which is present will have been spotted; it is nevertheless essential to proceed through the following steps, which involve a careful scrutiny using a magnifying glass and a bright light.

Step 5

Carefully inspect the skin and subcutaneous fat around the entire periphery of the breast image, looking for skin thickening, lack of definition of the deep surface of the skin and any excess of linear shadows traversing the fatty space between the breast tissue and the skin. It is important to compare the appearances at a site in one breast with those in the same position on the other side, before an appearance is judged to be abnormal (*Figure 6.4a, b*).

Step 6

Compare the nipples and subareolar regions:

- Is the nipple everted or indrawn?
- Are the subareolar ducts more prominent than usual?
- Are they the same on both sides?

Step 7

Inspect every square centimetre of both breasts looking for distortion of the normal parenchymal pattern, including, very importantly, any interruption of a linear shadow which may be present.

Step 8

Reinspect every square millimetre of both breasts using a magnifying lens in a search for calcifications (*Figure 6.5*).

Step 9

Look specifically at the axillary region of both sides to detect the presence of glands (*Figure 6.6*).

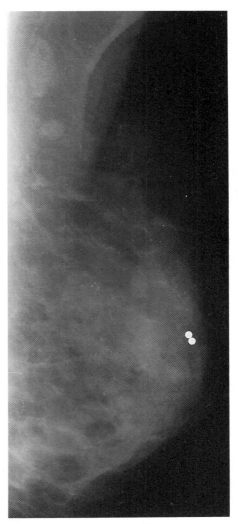

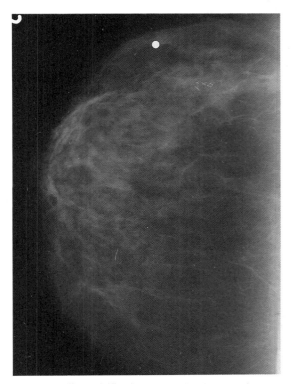

Figure 6.5 Microcalcification present in a 2-cm carcinoma

Figure 6.6 Glands noted in axilla

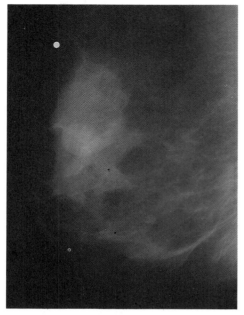

Figure 6.7 Rounded homogeneous lesion showing fibroadenoma

Step 10

If the reason has not already become obvious, go back to any area of asymmetry which was detected to see if a cause can now be identified.

Only now is one ready to progress to the stage of interpretation. It is not possible in a volume of this size to give exhaustive descriptions of all lesions – the reader should avail himself/herself of the assistance available in one of the several excellent atlases of mammographic appearances. However, there are several important signs which will assist in the elucidation of the mammographic abnormalities detected by the initial film reading exercise.

Interpretation of mass lesions

Texture

A homogeneous lesion is more likely to be benign than one which is non-homogeneous (*Figure 6.7*).

A lesion denser than the surrounding breast tissue is more likely to be malignant than one which is less dense.

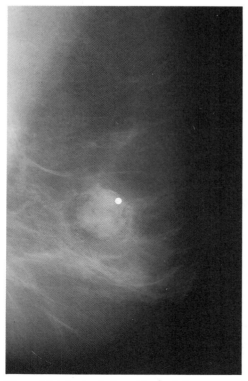

Figure 6.8 A benign lesion with a well demonstrated margin and a halo of fat

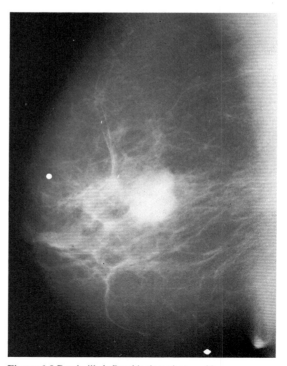

Figure 6.9 Partly ill-defined lesion obscured by parenchymal shadowing. This was a carcinoma

Margins

A benign lesion usually has a smooth, well-demarcated margin, often surrounded by the *halo of fat* it has displaced (*Figure 6.8*).

Smooth lobulation of the margin of a lesion suggests a fibroadenoma or a cluster of cysts.

If part of the *margin of a lesion is ill-defined*, it should be regarded as probably malignant. It is often difficult to be certain if a part of the margin is genuinely ill-defined, or if it is obscured by overlying parenchymal shadowing (*Figure 6.9*).

An *irregular spiculated margin* indicates a malignant lesion (*Figure 6.10*), particularly if the spicules are relatively short for the size of the lesion (*Figure 6.11*).

Location

A lesion which lies outside the involuted portion of the breast has a relatively high chance of being malignant (*Figure 6.12*).

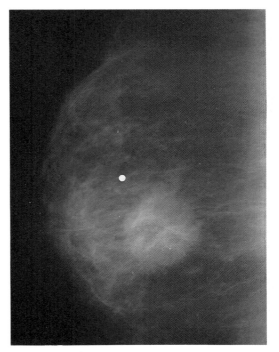

Figure 6.11 Spiculated malignant lesion (carcinoma)

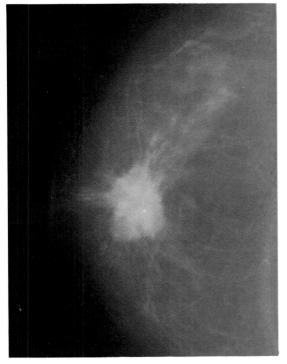

Figure 6.10 Spiculated malignant lesion (carcinoma)

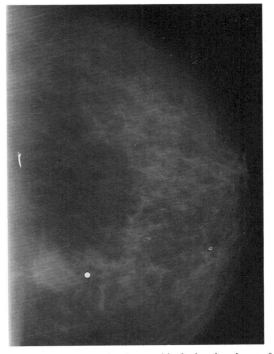

Figure 6.12 Carcinoma lying outside the involuted part of the breast

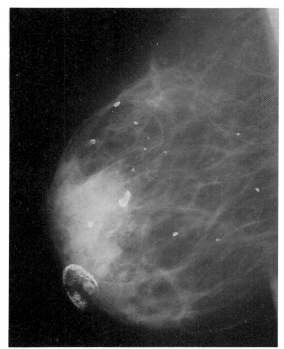

Figure 6.13 Coarse benign-type microcalcification and calcified oil cyst

Interpretation of calcifications

- Large (>1 mm diameter) coarse calcifications are likely to be benign (*Figure 6.13*).
- Single calcifications are likely to be benign.
- Rounded calcifications of equal size are likely to be benign.
- *Clusters of fine* calcifications are likely to signify malignancy (*Figure 6.14*).
- Rows of fine calcifications (in the ducts) are likely to signify malignancy.
- Short rods of *calcification, particularly if they branch*, are highly likely to signify malignancy (*Figure 6.15*).
- Groups of calcifications of mixed size with irregular shapes are more likely to signify malignant than benign disease.
- Calcifications scattered through both breasts are more likely to be associated with benign disease (*Figure 6.16a, b*).

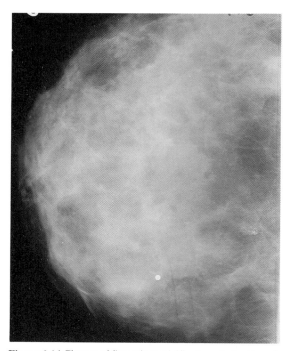

Figure 6.14 Cluster of fine microcalcifications indicative of malignant disease

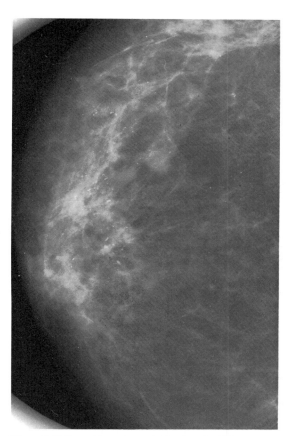

Figure 6.15 Branching microcalcification signifying malignancy

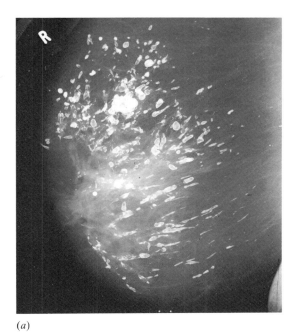

(a)

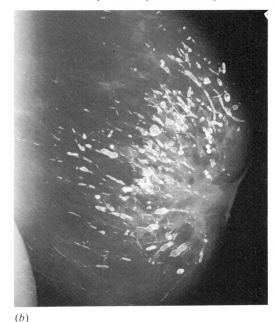

(b)

Figure 6.16 Coarse calcifications throughout both breasts

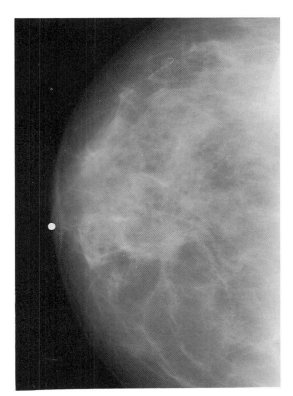

Figure 6.17 Parenchymal strands pulled in towards the lesion

Interpretation of parenchymal deformities

- If the parenchyma appears pushed aside by a lesion, the lesion is likely to be benign.
- If the parenchymal strands are pulled in towards a lesion it is more likely to be malignant (*Figure 6.17*).
- If parenchymal strands are actually interrupted by a lesion, it is highly likely to be malignant.

Interpretation of the reaction of a lesion

Subcutaneous reaction

This is the term given to an excess of linear shadows in the subcutaneous region seen adjacent to a superficial lesion passing right across to join the skin. When generalized, the reaction can be due to any one of a large number of causes, but when localized it is a highly significant marker suggesting malignancy (*Figure 6.18*).

Skin thickening

Localized skin thickening is virtually always associated with a fairly obvious subcutaneous reaction. The deep surface of the skin becomes slightly spiculated in the early stages and finally the

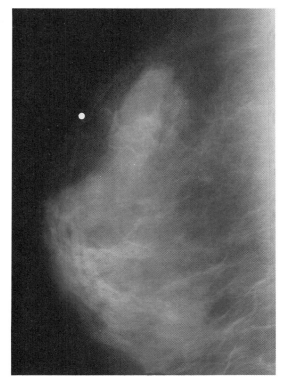

Figure 6.18 Subcutaneous reaction and underlying malignant lesion

thickened segment of the skin is drawn in towards the lesion. This strongly suggests malignancy (*Figure 6.19*).

Distant skin thickening may be observed secondary to lymphatic obstruction or to oedema produced by a lesion. It can best be observed inferior and medially and also in the periareolar region. When detected, it is a highly significant finding and the cause must be identified. Bilateral skin thickening can result from a generalized condition such as heart failure.

Prominent duct reaction

A leash of prominent ducts extending from a lesion towards the nipple strongly suggests malignancy (*Figure 6.20*), particularly if the leash has a biconvex appearance, converging both on the lesion and on the nipple. A fan-shaped leash of prominent ducts extending from the nipple is likely to be due to duct ectasia (*Figure 6.21*).

Oedema

An appearance of oedema is a difficult sign. It can be mimicked by inadequate compression or by unsharpness due to movement. When present,

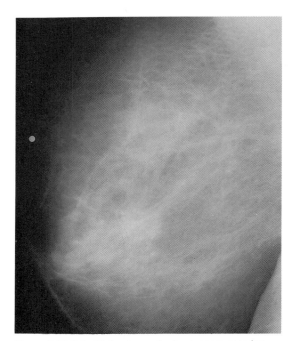

Figure 6.19 Skin thickening and subcutaneous reaction

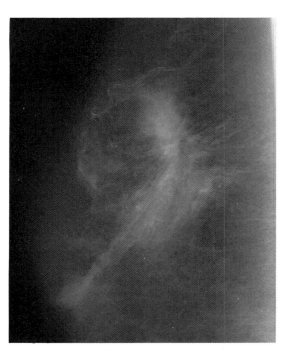

Figure 6.20 A leash of prominent ducts extending from the lesion towards the nipple

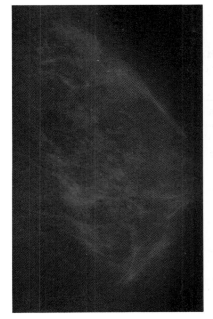

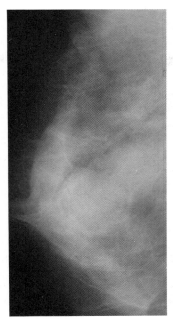

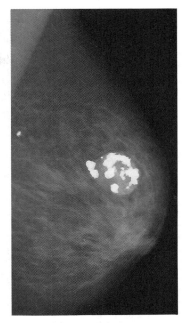

Figure 6.21 A fan leash of prominent ducts extending from the nipple

Figure 6.22 Multiple homogeneous densities representing cysts

Figure 6.23 Fibroadenoma with coarse 'popcorn' calcification

oedema is recognized by a slight diffuse increase in density which fades away to blend imperceptibly into the normal tissue. Within the affected area, the parenchymal strands are thickened with blurred margins. Commonly, but not necessarily, there is an associated subcutaneous reaction or skin thickening. Oedema signifies inflammatory disease, which may be actual infection (such as an abscess) or may be due to an active zone of dysplasia. Malignant lesions not uncommonly have a relatively narrow halo of oedema surrounding them.

In addition to the forgoing discussion of mammographic signs it is of value to list a few specific lesions and describe their characteristics.

Cysts (*Figure 6.22*)

- Often more than one.
- Commonly bilateral.
- Homogeneous.
- Smooth well-defined margins.
- The surface may calcify.

Fibroadenoma (*Figure 6.23*)

- Look like cysts, but may be lobulated.
- Characteristic coarse popcorn calcification occurs within them.

Carcinomas

- Dense spiculated lesions.
- Interrupt the parenchyma.
- Associated with microcalcifications.
- May present as microcalcifications alone.

Radial scar

A radial scar can very closely mimic a carcinoma, but classically will present as a lesion with a relatively radiolucent centre and very long spicules. Since radial scars are usually discoid in shape, they will appear larger and rounder on one view, and flattened on the other – unless by mischance both projections view the lesion from a similar angle (*Figure 6.24a, b*).

Sclerosing adenosis

- Usually a bilateral condition giving an increase in diffuse density and associated with microcalcifications (*Figure 6.25*). This microcalcification may be of the characteristic snowflake variety or may be identical to that associated with a carcinoma.
- When localized, sclerosing adenosis is absolutely indistinguishable from a carcinoma (*Figure 6.26*).

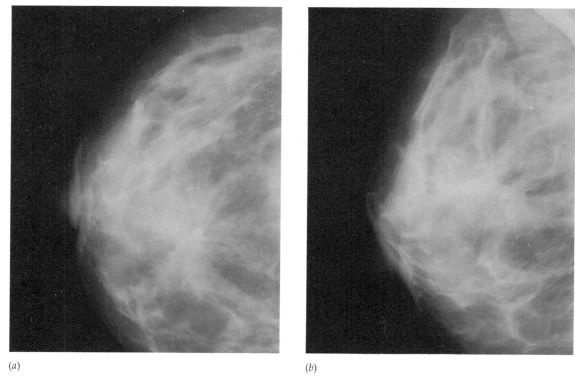

(a)   (b)

Figure 6.24 (a) Craniocaudal view showing radial scar; (b) 45° oblique view showing radial scar

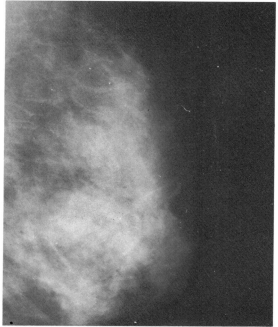

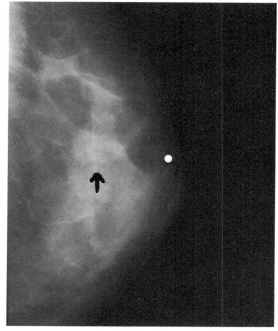

Figure 6.25 Scattered microcalcification in dense breasts indicative of sclerosing adenosis

Figure 6.26 Cluster of microcalcification in sclerosing adenosis which can mimic carcinoma

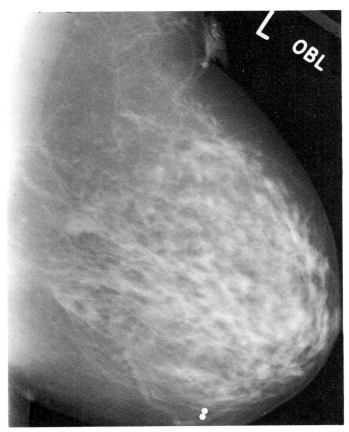

Figure 6.27 Duct dysplasia – a prominent duct pattern
(skin lesion also present)

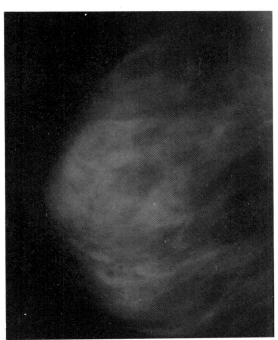

Figure 6.28 Gland dysplasia: honeycomb-like appearance,
often associated with multiple cysts

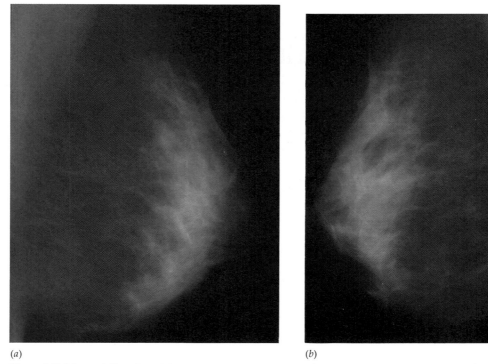

(a)   (b)

Figure 6.29 Bilateral dilatation of the main subareolar ducts showing duct ectasia

Epitheliosis

This may present an appearance very similar to sclerosing adenosis.

Mastitis/dysplasia

The two main varieties present mammographically:

1. Duct dysplasia – with prominent ducts throughout both breasts (*Figure 6.27*).

2. Gland dysplasia (fibroadenosis) which gives a honeycomb-like appearance, often associated with multiple cysts (*Figure 6.28*).

Duct ectasia

Dilatation of the main subareolar ducts is a fairly common occurrence, it is bilateral and, in the chronic stage, is associated with indrawing of the nipples. The dilated ducts may become secondarily infected giving a septic duct discharge (*Figure 6.29*).

7

Mammography – quality control and dose control

Quality control within a unit, and quality assurance between units, are equally important. There is, of course, some overlap between the two functions. In order to achieve the requisite high standards of mammography there should be involvement of radiologists, radiographers and physicists with a knowledge and interest in mammographic quality.

Quality assurance

Probably the most efficient way to establish a national and a regional quality assurance programme is to identify a series of reference centres, each with a number of satellite mammography units. In addition to the maintenance of the standards of existing equipment, some centres should undertake the testing of new equipment – mammographic machines, new film/screen combinations, cassettes. Each centre would be a base from which a physicist would operate, with responsibilities for dose measurement and apparatus operating parameters (kilovoltage peak and timer accuracy for example). Standard phantoms and film step wedges would be issued from the quality assurance centres, with results being monitored at both unit level and centrally.

The quality assurance reference centre should also have a quality 'trouble-shooting' role and be easily available to every unit.

Quality control in a unit

The importance of regular checking of apparatus, particularly film processors, is well known to all radiographers. In the field of mammography, there is much less latitude than in general radiography so that processor temperatures and replenishment times, for example, have to be very closely monitored.

To maintain a high standard of accuracy, radiographic positioning must be a major continuous responsibility of each radiographer in charge of a mammography unit.

Every newly installed piece of apparatus should be thoroughly checked, both in order to confirm that the performance is up to specification and to ensure that the exposure parameters are matched to those of other units in the area. This will necessitate checking the milovoltage peak settings, the X-ray beam quality, the automatic exposure control and importantly the focal spot which must be measured at the operating kilovoltage.

New processors require similar intensive checking with particular reference to the cycle time, chemistry temperature control and replenishment rates. Subsequently these items should be checked at regular intervals, say 6-monthly. At these inspections mechanical parts, for instance compression devices, should be checked for wear.

Dose monitoring is extremely important. Once the initial dose rates have been established by phantom measurements, the most convenient check is by a regular recording of the after-reading milliampere-seconds meter values.

Performance monitoring

In addition to technical quality aspects, it is necessary to monitor the performance of film readers, i.e. radiologists, clinic doctors or radiographers, and examine their actual reading technique.

This is a function which, while very necessary, is likely to be viewed with suspicion if not actual hostility by the professionals being monitored. Considerable tact is necessary in the setting up and operation of this performance monitoring. When it becomes known that everyone is being monitored, rather than just selected individuals, monitoring is regarded as much less of a 'witch hunt' and more of a helpful checking system. The accuracy of the basic film reading in a screening unit can be checked by sending on to an assessment team (*see* Chapter 10) a random sample of films classified as normal. In addition, a check can be performed by interposing films with known pathology among the films presented to the film reader.

With regard to radiographic positioning, it is likely that consistently higher standards will be achieved if a small panel of experienced practising radiographers regularly and formally reviews a random sample of the films taken in each unit.

Finally, in the case of screening units, one of the best indices of performance is the number of cancers identified per thousand cases examined, together with the size of the tumours at the time of detection.

8

Mammography – place in evaluation of the symptomatic patient

Should all patients complaining of breast symptoms have a mammogram? Ideally they should, as long as they are over the age of 35; the mammogram below that age is unlikely to be helpful because of the dense glandular nature of the breast tissue and because carcinoma below the age of 35 is rare. However, mammography is an expensive procedure (the average district general hospital would have to carry out some 2000 mammograms per year to cover all the symptomatic patients) and is counterproductive unless the technique is meticulous and there is local expertise in interpretation. At present these criteria are often unsatisfied in many district general hospitals. In addition there is a further danger: the interpretation by the referring doctor – that a negative mammogram means that no abnormality is present.

Mammography picks out around 85 per cent of symptomatic, palpable cancers, but the other 15 per cent are not visualized. Mammography also falsely identifies around three benign lesions as being possible cancers to every cancer that it detects (*Figure 8.1*).

A patient complaining of a breast symptom should be referred to a breast clinic, where there will first be an adequate clinical examination. After such an examination the reasons for carrying out mammography to aid diagnosis are (in women over 35):

1. At palpation the breasts do not feel entirely normal but there is no definite lump.
2. The complaint is of nipple discharge from a single duct (*see* Chapter 3).
3. Recent nipple indrawing, unless obviously benign on examination.
4. Eczema of the nipple has been found (*see* Chapter 3).
5. The complaint is of constant breast pain restricted to one area.
6. A lumpy area, but no definite lump, remains after draining a cyst (*see* Chapter 4).
7. After finding a cyst in a postmenopausal woman.
8. To ensure that an abscess has completely resolved (*see* Chapter 13).

Our recommendation for diagnosis of the symptomatic woman is to carry out a careful clinical examination and to act upon this as described in

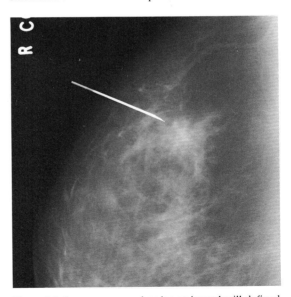

Figure 8.1 A mammogram showing an irregular ill-defined lesion mimicking cancer which is, in fact, benign on histology (sclerosing adenosis)

51

Chapter 4. There are clear indications for mammography in evaluation of the *symptomatic patient* and these should be remembered rather than using mammography in every patient. Mammography is of course the method of choice for *screening* and is also used to further evaluate the patient with *proven cancer* to determine whether the cancer is suitable for local excision (*see* Chapter 14), to *follow-up* the opposite breast and to *follow-up* the breast treated by local excision of the cancer and radiotherapy.

9

Other methods of imaging the breast

The standard method of breast imaging is by X-ray. Alternative methods or investigations which at present or in the future may provide an adjunct to clinical examination and mammography are:

1. Ultrasonography and Doppler ultrasound.
2. Transillumination.
3. Thermography and microwave thermography.
4. X-ray computerized tomography.
5. Magnetic resonance imaging.
6. Electric impedance.

Ultrasonography

The equipment used for ultrasound can be divided into two categories: static B scanners and real-time scanners.

Static B scanners produce static images of high degree resolution – usually the older type of equipment. Specialized units give high resolution images at intervals through the breast; the patient lies prone with the breast suspended in a water bath and multiple units then scan the breast with a large number of images produced. These units are highly specialized and expensive and are more popular abroad than in the UK.

Real-time scanners are more modern units which produce moving images; these can be of poorer resolution than static scanners. There are two types of real-time scanners: linear array and sector scanners. Linear array scanners produce a rectangular image with a large area of skin contact. Sector scanners produce a triangular image and have only a small area of skin contact. Real-time equipment is cheaper, more mobile, more versatile and easier to use than the static B scanner.

Grey scale ultrasound is imaging based on the amplitude of echoes returning from the tissues which determine whether masses are solid or cystic. A hand-held transducer with a frequency in the range of 5–9 MHz is directed at a specific location in the breast identified by palpation or by a specific finding on a mammogram; thus ultrasound is a second-line investigation and is not intended as a screening method. Ultrasound may be used by a radiographer to check an impalpable lesion he/she has seen on a mammogram and to give immediate confirmation (*Figure 9.1*) that the lesion is cystic. Also in more diffuse breast disease, ultrasound may be used as a back-up to conventional mammography and may show a solid lump amid the diffuse disease (*Figure 9.2a,b*). Impalpable lesions seen on mammograms can be localized by ultrasound for aspiration or biopsy as an alternative to mammographically guided marker-biopsy.

The disadvantages of ultrasound are that it has inadequate specificity in differentiating between different types of solid lesions, it is insensitive in investigating microcalcifications seen on mammography and the technique is time intensive. On the other hand, radiographers can be trained in the techniques required for its use in the immediate recognition of cysts and in placing aspiration needles for cytology.

In summary, grey scale ultrasonography of the breasts is a useful adjunct to mammography in the symptomatic woman, but is not considered suitable as the principal method for mass screening.

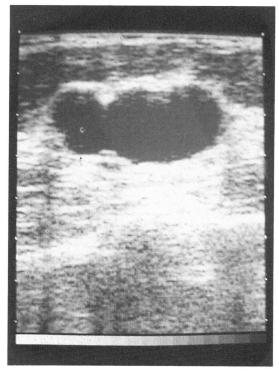

Figure 9.1 A breast cyst on ultrasound. A clear cyst with an area of enhancement behind it is seen

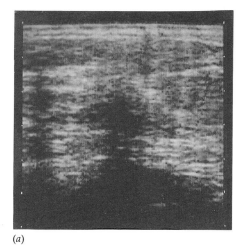

(a)

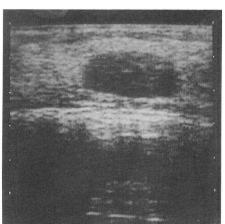

(b)

Figure 9.2 Solid lesions on ultrasound: (*a*) a carcinoma – irregular echo, poor mass with attenuation; (*b*) a fibroadenoma – well-defined echo, poor mass with a little enhancement

Doppler ultrasound

Doppler ultrasound is based on the detection of motion and is capable of demonstrating flow changes in the region of tumours related to the presence of tumour vessels. Pulsed Doppler, using duplex scanners, is currently being investigated to determine its role in breast diagnosis.

Transillumination – 'Lite-scan'

The basis for detecting abnormalities by 'Lite-scan' (Spectrascan Inc., Connecticut, USA) is the differential absorption and scattering of the light by the tissues. The transmitted light is directed via a video camera to an analogue-to-digital converter which processes the image and displays on a visual display unit (VDU) screen. Current Lite-scanners use visible red and infrared light pulsed sequentially through the breast using a hand-held light source (wand) placed against the breast (*Figure 9.3*). As the light passes through the tissues, it is reflected,

scattered and absorbed and the interaction of the two wavelengths in the tissues, the intensivity of the absorption, the appearance of absorptive areas, (*Figure 9.4*), variations in vascularity and variation of absorption in different parts of the spectrum provide information for diagnosis. Each breast is traditionally imaged in six different views (*Figure 9.5*) with the images recorded on video tape and floppy disk, which takes approximately 15–20 minutes per patient examination.

In Nottingham, we have assessed the diagnostic value of Lite-scanning in women with symptomatic breast disease by a commercially available Lite-scanner (Spectrascan Model 10). In 285 patients

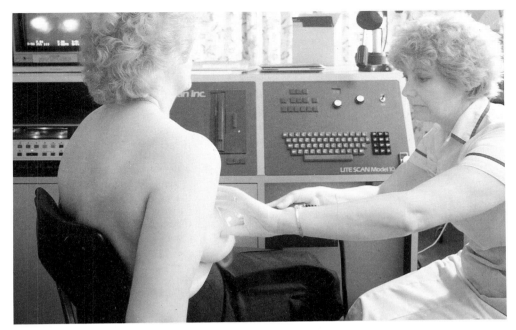

Figure 9.3 'Lite-scanning'

with symptomatic breast disease, with 41 cancers diagnosed, the results of Lite-scanning showed a sensitivity for cancer recognition of 87.8 per cent and a specificity of 71 per cent (*Table 9.1*). Of these

patients, 164 had both mammography and Lite-scan and 30 of these had breast cancers proven on biopsy; all 30 cancers were identified by either mammography or Lite-scan (*Table 9.2*). The sensitivity of

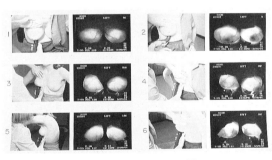

Figure 9.4 Carcinoma in right breast on Lite-scan

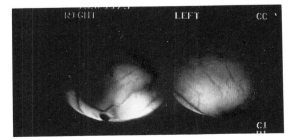

Figure 9.5 Imaging the breasts by Lite-scan

Table 9.1 Results of Lite-scan in 285 patients in the symptomatic referral clinic

Lite-scan report	*Benign*		*Malignant*
	Fibroadenoma	*Other*	
Malignant + indeterminate	14	56	36
Probably benign + normal	11 (all normal)	163	5

Sensitivity 36/41 = 87.8%.
Specificity 174/244 = 71.3%.

Table 9.2 Investigation of 30 carcinomas identified by mammography or Lite-scan

Lite-scan	*Mammography*	*No. of patients*
Positive	Positive	21
Positive	Negative	5
Negative	Positive	4

Lite-scan was as high as that of mammography – the specificity lower (*Table 9.3*). In other words, Lite-scanning identifies as many cancers as mammography in the symptomatic situation but picks out more breasts requiring investigation that ultimately prove benign.

Table 9.3 Comparison of sensitivity and specificity of mammography and Lite-scan in 164 cases of symptomatic breast disease imaged by both techniques

	Benign (*n* = 134)	Malignant (*n* = 30)
Reports of Lite-scan*		
Malignant + indeterminate (*n* = 70)	44	26
Probably benign + normal (*n* = 94)	90	4
Reports of mammography†		
Malignant + indeterminate (*n* = 55)	29	26
Probably benign + normal (*n* = 109)	105	4

* Sensitivity = 87%; specificity = 67%.
† Sensitivity = 87%; specificity = 78%.

Transillumination is non-invasive and non-ionizing and has high patient acceptability. When used in conjunction with clinical examination and mammography, Lite-scanning may help reduce the number of negative biopsies and has a high sensitivity for carcinoma. It is time intensive and is therefore not suitable for mass screening.

Our present investigation is to use Lite-scan-trained radiographers for the initial evaluation of the symptomatic breast by real-time Lite-scanning with palpation. We are evaluating whether this preliminary examination may improve the accuracy of diagnosis of breast cancer, reduce the number of mammograms required and reduce the number for follow-up examinations because of the confidence of the initial diagnosis.

Thermography

Thermography has been utilized in various forms:

1. Infrared thermography.
2. Liquid crystal thermography.
3. Computer-assisted thermography.
4. Microwave thermography.

All are based on the presumption that tumours emit more heat than the surrounding tissues. The basic technique has been in use for many years, but, with a few exceptions, conventional thermography is regarded as ineffective in detecting impalpable breast cancers either as a screening test or in a symptomatic population. The investigation is more operator dependent than any of the others.

Microwave thermography is a new method which examines emissions direct from a lesion rather than radiant heat rising from conducted heat to the skin. An early investigation of the method by a Glasgow team shows some promise. The method is easy to use and could in the future be applied by specially trained radiographers. The heat emission is measured at points at 2-cm intervals over the whole breast and from these a total picture is assembled.

X-ray computerized tomography

Breast lumps have been seen on CT investigation of the chest. However, for imaging the breast itself CT scanning is not used because of cost and time factors and irradiation dose. It could find a place as a second-line investigation of mammographically identified lesions.

Magnetic resonance imaging

Magnetic resonance imaging (MRI) is a new diagnostic imaging technique which may give additional tissue characteristics. MRI scanners involve multiplanar tomographic imaging. Using specially developed radiofrequency antennae (surface coil), high resolution MR images of the breast can be obtained without ionizing radiation. A wide variety of breast morphology can be imaged; fat, gland and fibrous tissues can be identified (*Figure 9.6*).

In general, malignant tumours show excellent contrast with surrounding fatty tissues on T1 weighted images, because on these images tumours have decreased signal while fat shows a markedly intense signal. MRI demonstrates great potential in imaging the breast and newer developments may increase the specificity and give better tissue characterization. However, it is very time consuming to image the whole breast. MRI could be developed to further investigate lesions seen on mammography but it is not a first-line screening tool.

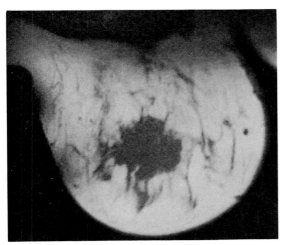

Figure 9.6 MRI of the breast using surface coils. A large low intensity mass is seen in the centre of the breast and fibrous septa are displayed as low intensity linear structures within the high intensity tissue

Applied potential tomography: electric impedance

This is in the very early stages of development. A series of electrodes is placed on the surface of the breast and a small constant electrical current is applied in sequence between pairs of electrodes; any impedance in the current is measured in ohms. The overall picture is obtained by computerized tomography.

Conclusion

At present mammography is the established method of investigation after clinical examination of symptomatic women and in particular is the accepted method for population screening. Real-time ultrasound is useful to instantly differentiate lesions into benign cysts requiring no further investigation and solid lesions.

Of the other methods at present under investigation, Lite-scanning is promising and its usefulness may be as a real-time method combined with palpation in the initial assessment of the symptomatic patient. MRI gives a good image of the breast tissue, it is time intensive and costly at present, but may ultimately provide the most accurate back-up to examine mammographically detected lesions. Microwave thermography is still at the research stage but might provide an alternative screening method.

10

The early detection of breast cancer and mammographic screening

The logical basis for early detection is that a woman who has a breast cancer removed when it is small has a much better chance of long-term survival than a woman with a large breast cancer. However, this could be a simplistic argument, because slow growing cancers, which would do well anyway because they are well differentiated (*see* Chapter 1), spend longer at a small size and are more likely to be detected then. To test whether breast cancer screening is effective it was necessary to run clinical trials.

HIP study

The Health Insurance Plan trial (HIP) in New York was a randomized trial involving 62 000 women aged 40–64, and included examination by a surgeon and two-view mammography. Screening was carried out annually for 4 years only. The acceptance rate was low, only 40 per cent attended on four screenings, 53 per cent attended two or more and only 65 per cent attended even one screening.

The number of cancers diagnosed in the study population was virtually the same as the number diagnosed in the control population (*Table 10.1*): this figure suggests that every case that was diagnosed as cancer in the study group would have turned into a clinical breast cancer.

The crucial figure is that mortality from breast cancer was cut by one-third in the population invited for screening (*Table 10.1*). Mortality figures are a very hard statistic – there is no explanation for this finding other than that screening saved women from dying from breast cancer. In the HIP programme,

Table 10.1 Deaths from breast cancer in the HIP study at 5 years and at 14 years from the start of the programme

	Number	No. of deaths from breast cancer	
		At 5 years	At 14 years
Study	306	39	118
Control	300	63	153

even at 18 years, there remains a significant difference in mortality from breast cancer. An even greater reduction in mortality might have been achieved if more people had attended for screening.

Case survival graphs (*Figure 10.1*; the follow-up of patients with cancer) show that the group with the best prognosis after diagnosis was that in which the cancers were detected at the screening examination by mammography.

The Swedish Study of Kopperberg and Ostergotland Counties is very different in method. This consists of a single view oblique mammography every 2–3 years, with no clinical examination, and is therefore a cost-effective programme. It is a randomized trial of women aged 40–74, and the randomization deliberately included more women in the study group (78 085) than in the control group (56 782). Attendance rates were very high: 90–95 per cent. Again there is a one-third diminution in mortality from breast cancer up to 9 years of study (*Figure 10.2*); no difference was found in the 40- to 49-year-olds (*Table 10.2*) but for the older women in the study group there were, by 5 years, 71 breast

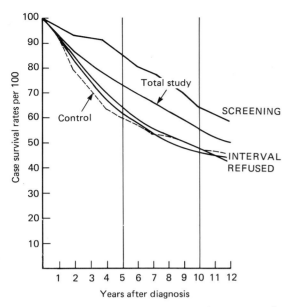

Figure 10.1 Graphs of case survival drawn from reports of the HIP study. Top line: patients with cancers diagnosed at screening examinations (usually by mammography). Other lines: control population; screened population – cancers diagnosed between screening examinations; screened population – non-attenders after invitation for screening

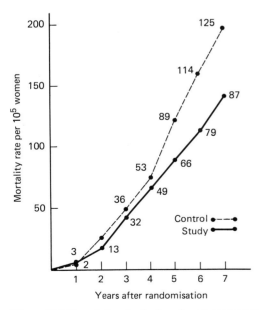

Figure 10.2 Cumulative deaths from breast cancer per 100 000 women in the Swedish screening study. (From Tabar, Gad *et al.* (1985) Reduction in mortality from breast cancer after mass screening with mammography. *The Lancet*, pp. 829–832. Reproduced by kind permission of *The Lancet*)

Table 10.2 Deaths from breast cancer in the Swedish study at 5 years from the start of the programme

	Deaths from breast cancer	
40–49 age group		
Study	16 in 19 938 women	} NS
Control	10 in 15 678 women	
50–74 age group		
Study	71 in 58 148 women	} $P<0.003$
Control	76 in 41 104 women	

cancer deaths in nearly 60 000, and in the control groups slightly more cancer deaths in only just over 40 000 women.

Screening a population results in a very high initial pick-up rate at the very first screening; the excess breast cancers are those which would normally have presented clinically over the following months. In Guildford and in Edinburgh the number of *in situ* cancers (*see* Chapter 2) being detected is around the 20 per cent level, whereas the normal presentation without screening is around 3 per cent. This pick-up of *in situ* cancers may in part explain the success of screening.

Mammographic screening does, however, have its problems, the overriding one being that of cost. The reason for this is that the incidence of breast cancer is only between one and two per thousand women each year. The benign biopsy rate can be frightening – this arises from mammographic abnormalities which are due to benign changes. The benign-to-malignant biopsy ratio can only be kept to a reasonable level if there is expertise in taking and reading mammograms, good back-up (such as magnification), a clear policy for indeterminate lesions (*see* Chapter 12) and regular decision-making meetings with a surgeon. The possibility of the false diagnosis of breast cancer arises from two lesions: sclerosing adenosis and radial scar (*see* Chapters 2 and 6). Mammographically these closely mimic cancer and, unfortunately, sclerosing adenosis might be interpreted as cancer by the unwary pathologist. Entrenched medical attitudes must change to allow superspecialization to give expertise and to enable close cooperation between radiographer, pathologist, radiologist and surgeon to facilitate the running of effective screening programmes.

There are two ways of minimizing costs: to introduce low cost mammography or low cost physical examination and to use selective factors. Palpation by an external observer should be ruled out as ineffective and costly. All physical methods require an operator and this is where their cost lies; mammography is not likely to be replaced by any other physical method for some time to come (*see* Chapter 9). No selective factors are yet strong enough to base screening programmes upon them.

At what age should screening start? *Figure 10.3* shows the age incidence for cancer in the Nottingham series. There is a sharp increase at the age of

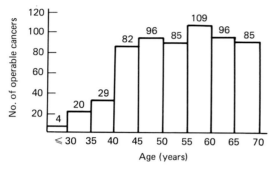

Figure 10.3 Age incidence of 606 cancers in the Nottingham series (up to age 70)

40–45. Below 40 breast cancer comes to only one woman in 10 000 each year. Programmes cannot be extended to the under-forties, which would not only be highly cost-inefficient but also would result in picking up much benign disease and carrying out of unnecessary benign biopsies. There is, in fact, no good evidence from the trials that screening succeeds below the age of 50 and this may be a reflection of the difficulties in reading the denser mammogram below that age.

Breast self-examination (BSE) is cheap, more efficient than examination by an external observer and should probably be added to mammographic programmes (*see* Chapter 11), because one-third to one-half of breast cancers will still present in the intervals between screenings.

Table 10.3 compares the costs for breast self-examination, annual single-view mammography,

biennial single-view mammography and annual two-view plus clinical examination as carried out in the New York HIP study. This does not include secondary costs such as the cost of biopsy.

Annual costs for the average health district, with 30 000 women at risk, come to £14 000 for BSE and self-referral, £70 000 for the Swedish style screening (biennial single-view oblique mammography), £100 000 for annual single-view and £200 000 for two-view and clinical examination. We recommend a combination of biennial single view without clinical examination but with the addition of BSE. Swedish figures have shown that this type of screening can be performed very efficiently and the results are nearly as good as two-view mammography with clinical examination. There is some evidence to support BSE and the need for this could be reinforced at each attendance for biennial mammography. *Table 10.3* shows the cost per carcinoma diagnosed per life saved. (Of five patients with breast cancer, at present one survives, one dies from other causes and three of breast cancer. Since screening appears to save one in three who die from the disease, it will therefore save one in five of those who develop the disease.) This latter is the benefit to be set against the cost of screening.

Mammography for the symptomatic woman is often very badly used at the present time (*see* Chapter 8). Our drug bill for chemotherapy is enormous and the effect of chemotherapeutic agents in breast cancer is poor. Money could be saved from these areas of breast disease investigation and treatment and diverted to mammography screening.

The Department of Health, faced with some demand to implement screening, set up a committee chaired by Professor Sir Patrick Forrest, to consider the evidence for and the likely cost of screening. The 'Forrest' report (Department of Health and Social Security, *Breast Cancer Screening*, Report to the Health Ministers, HMSO) was accepted by the Government as the basis for the implementation of the national programme of screening women aged 50–64. This will be nationwide over the next 4 years and will rely upon 3-yearly mammograms by the single-view oblique technique. There will be local variations on the exact methods adopted within these broad outlines.

To set up the programme four teaching centres have been established in England (Guildford Jarvis Screening Centre, Nottingham City Hospital Helen Garrod Screening Unit, King's College Hospital and Manchester Withington Hospital; Edinburgh and Cardiff will be the teaching centres in Scotland and Wales).

Table 10.3 Costs of screening by different methods per cancer diagnosed, per life saved and per woman per annum

	BSE (£)	Single view		Two-view and clinical (£)
		Annual (£)	Biennial (£)	
Per cancer diagnosed	330	2222	1555	4523
Per cancer affected (1 in 5)	1650	11 109	7775	22 617
Per head per annum	0.49	3.33	2.30	6.78

11

Breast self-examination

For the last 7 years breast self-examination (BSE) has been under evaluation in Nottingham as part of the National Trial for Early Breast Cancer Detection.

BSE is easy to teach, easy to do and women examining their own breasts can find very small lumps and notice early changes in the appearance of the breasts. Teaching women BSE is obviously a much cheaper method of early breast cancer detection than mammographic screening.

Out of women within the age range 40–60 years in Nottingham, 89 010 were invited by personal letter over their general practitioner's name to attend a lecture on BSE; 37 788 attended giving an attendance rate of 42 per cent. The number of inaccuracies in the Family Practitioner Committee records gives a corrected attendance of greater than 50 per cent for those women who received their invitations.

Lectures are held in, or close to, two self-referral units where women may refer themselves without prior consultation with their GPs if they subsequently find an abnormality. One of these units, the Helen Garrod Breast Screening Unit at the City Hospital, is staffed by specially trained radiographers. The other unit at the General Hospital is staffed by nursing sisters. The lectures on BSE are given by the radiographers and nursing sisters and consist of a short talk and film, with ample time for questions. Each woman is given a leaflet to take home reinforcing the message with the telephone number of the self-refer units, which she is encouraged to contact if she finds an abnormality.

When a woman subsequently self-refers she is examined by the same radiographers or nurses who gave the lectures and a two-view mammogram is taken. If the clinical examination is normal and the mammogram appears clear to the radiographer then the woman is discharged that day. A real-time ultrasound machine is available to the radiographers to ascertain whether an opacity on a mammogram, with no lump palpable, is in fact a cyst. Mammograms are later checked each week by the radiologist. An abnormality on clinical examination or on the mammogram results in a recall for assessment by the clinic doctor – one of the surgeons on the breast cancer unit. The clinic doctor drains any cysts and discharges the patient, takes a biopsy in the clinic of any solid lump and keeps under review any patients in whom there is no definite clinical or mammographic lesion but who are not found quite normal.

Looking at the pattern of work at the two units in the first 7 years since the scheme began, 89 010 were invited for lectures and 6852 self-referred subsequently. Of these, 4337 (63 per cent) were reassured and discharged at first visit when clinical examination and mammogram were judged normal by the radiographer; a further 514 had cysts aspirated and were discharged; 565 received biopsies, giving the final diagnosis as 274 cancers and 291 benign lesions – a cancer:benign ratio of 1:1.2.

If a patient has neither a definite clinical nor mammographic abnormality but one of them is not completely normal, then she is kept under review; it is our review policy to clinically re-examine at 2-monthly intervals and to re-mammogram at 6 months.

In all, 1446 patients have been kept under review at units in this fashion; 1385 were discharged at 6 months and some patients had cysts aspirated during that time and were discharged. Sixty-one biopsies were performed giving 16 cancers, 12 of these being small or *in situ* cancers diagnosed during the 6-month observation period; the delay would not seem to have adversely affected the outlook. In Nottingham, we have compared all the cancers arising in our study population in both districts with a group of historical controls.

1. *The study population* is the women invited for education from 1979 onwards and in which a breast cancer was subsequently diagnosed (*n* = 751).
2. *Control population* – same number of cancers (*n* = 751) in the age-matched population in the same health district, diagnosed immediately prior to the start of the education programme, i.e. the 751 cancers working chronologically backwards from the date education commenced.

Comparison of the two groups has been made of size of tumour at presentation, lymph node involvement at operation and of survival.

Women in the study group have more small tumours among the operable cancers and more patients are presenting without lymph node involvement. Thus prognostic features in the study group are more favourable (*Table 11.1*). Although there is no difference in survival between the two groups demonstrated in the early results at 7 years, it appears from the prognostic features that longer follow-up will result in a modest survival advantage.

An important part of the self-referral units is the quick, efficient treatment of the majority of self-referring women who can be relieved of their anxiety, reassured and discharged.

We recommend breast self-examination teaching with self-referral as an adjunct to a mammographic screening programme. Mammography alone will not diagnose all breast cancers, the usual sensitivity being quoted as 85–90 per cent and this inevitably means some breast cancers will be missed, while others will truly arise between screenings. BSE as a supplement will help to detect those interval cancers at an earlier stage. BSE teaching may also offer an important medicolegal protection to mammographic screening programmes, for women must be told that screening does not detect all cancers and women must still report symptoms as early as possible.

In mounting the programme of BSE with a self-referral clinic for back-up, radiographers have played a prominent and most responsible part. They carry out the lecture sessions, have shown themselves to be most adept at examination of the breast and have taken the clinical responsibility of deciding whether the breast is normal or not, produce mammograms of high quality and show high sensitivity in reading these.

Table 11.1 Cancers detected in the study and control populations

	Good prognosis	Moderate prognosis	Poor prognosis
Study (*n* = 395)	143 36%	195 49%	57 14%
Control (*n* = 286)	78 27%	135 47%	73 26%

$\chi^2 = 14.9$; 2 d.f.; $P < 0.001$.
Good prognosis: Patients with small or *in situ* cancers with lymph node negative at operation and with low histological grade.
Poor prognosis: Large or advanced tumours with node positive at operation and more agressive high grade tumours.

12

The organization of a screening service

It now appears that the mortality from breast cancer can be reduced by screening a population and thus detecting the disease at an early stage (*see* Chapter 10). Moreover, early detection increases the potential for treatment by conservative surgical measures rather than by mastectomy.

Identification of the population

The first step is to identify the population to be screened. Age is the most important risk factor for the development of breast cancer. The disease is rare below the age of 35, with an incidence of about 20 per 100 000 women; by the age of 50 years the incidence is nearly 150 per 100 000 women. Over the age of 65, women's response to invitations to be screened falls dramatically. It is for this reason that, as a first step, the age group of 50–65 years has been suggested for screening in the UK. As evidence accumulates, it is possible that screening at an earlier age may well be shown to be effective and the screening programme will need to be broadened to include these women.

The invitation

In order to obtain a high response rate, and thus increase the effectiveness of the screening programme, it has been shown in the Nottingham BSE programme (*see* Chapter 11) that women are more likely to accept a personalized invitation from their own general practitioner than from other sources. A response rate in the order of 70 per cent may be anticipated with a combination of personalized invitation and national publicity.

The basic screen

All women accepting the invitation will undergo the basic screening test (*Figure 12.1*) – in this context a single oblique mammogram of each breast (with the exception that on the first attendance both oblique and craniocaudal projections are recommended).

It goes without saying that the technical quality at this stage is of paramount importance to the success of the whole screening programme, positioning and film processing being the most important features (*see* Chapter 5). These are the province of the radiographer.

The mammograms are displayed ready for film *reading*, a multiviewer being preferred in order to cope with the large numbers involved. The object of the film reading process is to divide the films into those which are normal and those which are not absolutely normal. Film reading may be undertaken by one individual, but it has been shown that with two individuals reading the films on separate occasions a higher sensitivity is achieved, i.e. there are fewer false negatives or films wrongly consi-

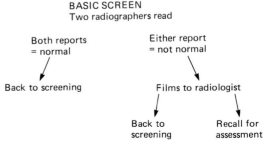

Figure 12.1 The screening procedure

63

dered to be normal in women with cancer. Radiographers, regularly taking and looking at mammograms, are probably the best group to undertake this initial read.

With non-radiologists (either doctors or radiographers) employed in film reading, some 20 per cent of films are likely to be judged 'not entirely normal'. These films are then interpreted by a radiologist experienced in mammography who will consider that a quarter to a half of them (5–10 per cent of the total screened) are sufficiently abnormal to merit referral of the women to the next stage – assessment.

Assessment

An expert multidisciplinary team is required at this stage (*Figure 12.2*): a radiologist, surgeon closely working with a pathologist, and an experienced radiographer.

In the assessment clinic, the woman has a clinical examination by the surgeon and any further mammographic views which may be required are taken. These commonly include rotated craniocaudal and lateral projections and often magnification views of a suspect area especially for microcalcification. It is also valuable to repeat the initial oblique view, because a slight variation in projection may prove that an original appearance of a lesion was in fact due to a summation shadow. Ultrasound examination may help in elucidation of a mammographic abnormality. Fine needle aspiration for cytology or Trucut biopsy of palpable abnormalities is undertaken. Increasingly, aspiration cytology will be used by a stereotactic technique for impalpable lesions.

Finally, a case conference between the experts involved will lead to a decision on each woman. The decision will be *either* that the woman is in fact normal (some 95 per cent of those recalled to the assessment clinic), requires a period of follow-up

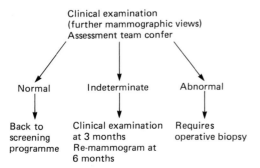

Figure 12.2 Assessment procedure

(re-mammogram after 6 months with interim clinical examinations), *or* that there is sufficient suspicion of cancer to merit an operative biopsy (or that cytology or Trucut biopsy in the assessment clinic has already confirmed the diagnosis of cancer).

Formal biopsy

The final stage before treatment is carried out is to make a firm diagnosis, although this will hopefully have been established in the assessment clinic. In the first screening round of the women originally screened, about 1–2 per cent will need biopsy or cytology in order to make a firm histological diagnosis and, of these, one-third to one-half of these will have breast cancer. The importance of the assessment clinic is in keeping down the number of operative biopsies either by confirming the diagnosis of cancer in the assessment clinic *or* by showing that biopsy is not necessary for a benign lesion. This is the reason why 'experts' regularly practising in breast disease need to staff the assessment clinic.

Screening interval

The ideal interval between attendances for screening examinations is unknown. Many trials in the past have arbitrarily chosen an interval of 1 year. The Swedish study has shown that substantial benefit can be achieved with a screening interval of nearly 3 years and, based on this evidence, a 3-year interval seems a reasonable starting point for a UK screening programme. However, there are results based on size and stage of detection which suggest that intervals of 18 months might be more effective, particularly in younger women.

Management and administration

In order to facilitate the smooth functioning of the system outlined above, it is essential that there is firm management – preferably by a working member of the screening team – and adequate clerical and administrative back-up.

Two important aspects of the organization merit specific mention. There must be prompt communication at all stages with both the patient and the general practitioner. Equally important, there must be an in-built fail-safe mechanism so that women considered to have a likelihood of cancer following the screening examinations do not by some mischance fail to be recalled to the next stage.

13

The management of benign breast conditions

Benign breast 'disease' is difficult to define. There are palpable lumps – cysts and fibroadenomas. These in themselves are not harmful and the only point of them is that they form a breast lump and any breast lump has to be fully diagnosed in case it is a cancer. Then there is breast pain, a symptom not a 'disease', for if the painful breast were to be inspected histologically it would appear like a normal breast, allowing for age.

Each condition does present a problem and this chapter describes the management of fibroadenoma, cyst (particularly recurrent and multiple cysts), abscess, mammillary fistula, breast pain, adenosis of pregnancy and phyllodes tumour (*see* Chapter 2).

Fibroadenoma

The clinical features have been described in Chapter 3, the pathology in Chapter 2, diagnosis in Chapter 4 and the mammographic features in Chapter 6.

Fibroadenoma is most common below the age of 30, when breast cancer is very uncommon (*see Figure 10.4*). Our management policy revolves round this fact.

A woman of up to 30, presenting with a small, very mobile, solid lump in the breast is investigated by fine needle aspiration (FNA) cytology (*see* Chapter 4) and the size of the lump is recorded. She is told that she may have the lump removed if she prefers to. Otherwise the policy is to carry out aspiration for cytology on two separate occasions 6 weeks apart. As long as both show epithelial cells in adequate numbers and these appear benign, then

the lump can be safely left. Most fibroadenomas remain static, a few increase in size; we therefore tell the patient to return if her lump grows.

If these criteria are not obeyed, i.e. the cells appear somewhat abnormal (as they may in fibroadenomas) or insufficient numbers of epithelial cells are present in the FNA, then the lump is removed. In a woman over 30 at present, the lump is removed for full histological examination in any case; in the future we may modify this policy and apply that used in the younger woman.

Cyst

As discussed in Chapter 4 the first diagnostic procedure for most breast lumps is to needle them. If the lump proves to be a cyst on needling, then it is aspirated completely. The examiner checks that no residual lump is present and, assuming this is so, then no further appointment is made for the patient.

Occasionally, the patient has to make frequent visits to the clinic because she is forming multiple palpable cysts. Each time she has a lump it has to be needled to make sure it is a cyst. We advise patients who are bothered by multiple recurrent cysts to try a 3-month course of danazol (Danol, Winthop Sterling; this drug is described in more detail under Breast pain). Both on palpation and mammographically (*Figures 13.1* and *13.2*), the number of cysts recurring are reduced and, even though the course lasts only 3 months, the reduction in the presentation of cysts is apparent 1 year later (*Table 13.1*).

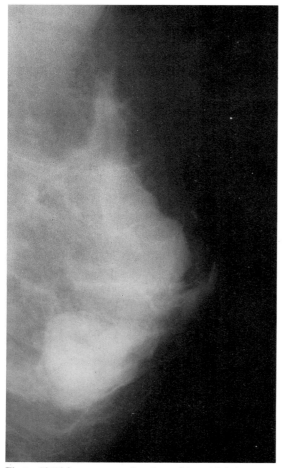

Figure 13.1 Mammogram of patient with multiple breast cysts before treatment with danazol

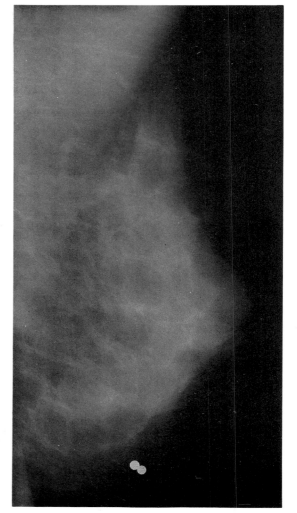

Figure 13.2 Mammogram of patient in *Figure 13.1* after treatment with danazol

Abscess

Abscess presents as an extremely tender, hot, red lump in the breast. It may be very large – around 10 cm diameter.

Breast abscesses occur in pregnancy and during lactation. They are treated like any other abscess – incised if fluctuant or causing a high fever or aborted with antibiotics if found early in their course.

When a breast abscess occurs outside pregnancy or lactation, we ensure that it has not arisen within any other pathology such as a cancer. The lump is observed until it has entirely disappeared; a mammogram is then taken. As long as this also is clear no further action is taken.

Table 13.1 Clinical requirement for cyst aspiration up to 6 months in the treated and control groups

Group	n	Cysts aspirated
Control	15	56
Danazol treated	18	35

Mammillary fistula

This is a condition giving rise to multiple or recurrent abscesses, around the edge of the areola (*Figure 13.3*). They are smaller and have more chronic courses than the acute abscess described above.

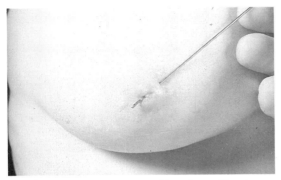

Figure 13.3 Mammillary fistula: this patient suffered a periareola abscess which discharged leaving an unhealed area. The probe has been passed through this into the duct from where the fistula is arising and out through the nipple. Treatment will be to incise along the probe and allow the fistula to granulate up

The pathology is that of duct ectasia (*see* Chapter 2) – infection arises in dilated ducts close to the nipple. The abscess bursts through to the skin leaving a fistula from duct to skin. This reopens when the infection arises again or may stay open with a chronic purulent discharge emerging through a point on the edge of the areola.

The initial treatment is to open the abscess down to the duct, place a probe in the duct and cut the duct open to the end of the nipple. The wound is not resutured but is allowed to slowly heal.

If this does not succeed, or other abscesses arise around the areola, then a cut is made around the lower half of the areola, the nipple is dissected from the deeper tissue and the central part of the whole duct system lying below the nipple and areola is removed.

Breast pain

Some breast discomfort associated with the premenstrual days is the normal condition; some women suffer no discomfort, the majority a little, some much more discomfort and a few genuine cyclical breast pain.

The majority of women who come to the breast referral clinic with the complaint of breast pain (300

of the 1700 patients attending the referral clinic in 1979) have come for reassurance that breast cancer is not the underlying cause. This is usually simple to give, because breast pain is rarely a symptom of primary breast cancer and all the breast cancers we have seen presenting as breast pain have also had a palpable breast lump.

This leaves a minority (around 60 of the 300) who are getting pain severe enough to make a difference to their life and thus require specific treatment for the pain itself.

In deciding upon treatment of these women the first essential is to clarify the type of breast pain.

Cyclical breast pain

This builds up to climax in the premenstrual week, is relieved when menstruation begins, is present for 3 weeks out of 4 restarting around 1 week after menstruation. The breast is tender and this may interfere with the woman's sex life. It is often associated with very lumpy breasts to palpation in the premenstrual week.

Cervical nerve root syndrome

Here the patient complains of non-cyclical pain in the lateral side of the breast or both breasts. On questioning she admits to pain also radiating to the arm, with paraesthesiae in the arm and often pain over the shoulder. X-ray of the neck may show cervical spondylitis (*see Figure 3.1*).

The cause of the pain is nerve root irritation due to disc or bone disease of the vertebral column. The treatment is initially by exercise to improve the muscles around the neck and shoulder girdle. If this fails then the patient is given physiotherapy.

Tietze's syndrome (limited fibromyalgia syndrome)

This is non-cyclical pain over the cartilaginous parts of the anterior ends of the ribs where they join the sternum. The exact pathology is not known. It is recognized by palpating with the fingers under the breast so that one is rubbing the costal cartilages themselves and comparing this with gently pinching the breast tissue; the former reproduces the patient's tenderness.

Treatment is by injecting local anaesthetic and hydrocortisone around the painful ribs.

Trigger spot

This is continuous pain and tenderness restricted to one area of the breast. Here a mammogram should be carried out to ensure that there is no underlying lesion. If none is demonstrated and the pain is bad enough, then exision of the painful area is curative of pain in around 50 per cent of cases.

Adenosis of pregnancy

This is a large lump (often 5–10 cm in diameter) in the already lumpy breast of pregnancy. The differential diagnosis is breast cancer. Adenosis is not a pathological entity and biopsy shows only breast tissue with the normal changes of pregnancy.

Presented with a pregnant patient with such a lump in the breast, our diagnostic procedure is to take Trucut biopsies (*see* Chapter 4) from opposite ends of the lump on two occasions 2 weeks apart. As long as all these show only normal breast tissue with pregnancy changes, we are confident that the lump is not malignant and we simply observe it until it resolves after lactation.

Phyllodes tumour

This is a tumour (*Figure 13.4*) that is usually benign (*see* Chapter 2). A smooth, sometimes lobulated, often large lump without any fixity occurring in a patient in the 60+ age group should make one think of phyllodes tumour (*see Figure 2.21*), since large

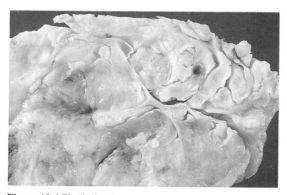

Figure 13.4 Phyllodes tumour

carcinomas usually show skin or deep fixity or *peau d'orange* of the overlying skin.

Diagnosis is made on Trucut biopsy; there are mammographic features of this tumour (*see* Chapter 6).

Treatment is to remove the tumour, usually by mastectomy. Occasionally these tumours show malignant features on histology and then a wide mastectomy is required as there is a high chance of local recurrence.

Mondor's sign

Occasionally, a superficial vein in the breast may clot, giving a cord-like feel and some mild discomfort; most often this is in a vein running from bottom to top in the lateral half of the breast. The thrombosis is accompanied by skin tether (*Figure 13.5*); this is known as Mondor's sign.

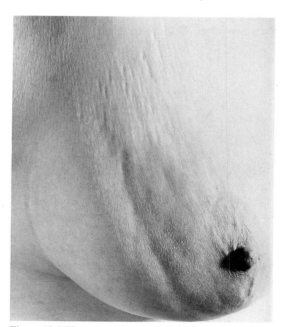

Figure 13.5 Thrombosis in a superficial vein giving longitudinal skin tether. Under this lies a cord-like thrombosed vein

14

Treatment of primary breast cancer

The 'primary' is the initial cancerous lump which has arisen in the breast (*Figure 14.1*).

Once a breast cancer has been diagnosed the patient requires definitive treatment. Treatment has two aims: possible cure of the patient and local control at the site of the primary growth.

As described in Chapter 2, many patients already have distant spread of their cancer by the time they are diagnosed and therefore 'cure' is not possible. However, about one in five will be a long-term survivor and one in three will die of something other than their breast cancer; in these 'cure' can be achieved and is worth striving for.

Even if the patient dies from distant spread, every effort should be made to ensure that they do not also suffer the discomfort of an uncontrolled cancer on the chest wall (*Figure 14.2*).

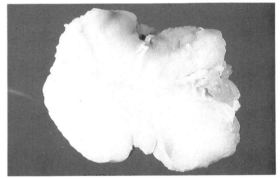

Figure 14.1 A primary carcinoma in the operative specimen

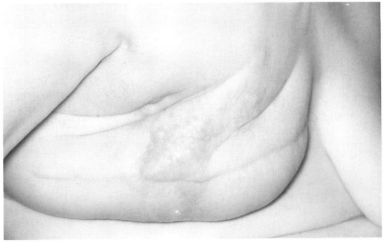

Figure 14.2 A local recurrence within the mastectomy flaps

To best achieve these aims the accepted rule is that the whole breast requires treatment. A number of breast cancers arise in more than one site in the breast and removal of the diagnosed lump alone would not be sufficient in those patients. Furthermore, in a large series carried out in the USA, recurrence within the breast occurred in 40 per cent of patients who had their cancerous lump alone removed without further treatment.

The traditional method of treatment is by mastectomy but there are now alternatives.

Mastectomy

The operation accepted by the majority of surgeons in the UK as suitable treatment for invasive breast cancer is simple mastectomy. This operation involves a transversely placed elliptical incision around the palpable mass in the breast, including the nipple and areola.

The surgeon dissects under the skin flaps so that, together with the skin ellipse, he is able to remove all the breast tissue down to the pectoral muscle, dissecting almost up to the clavicle and removing the axillary tail of the breast. The skin ellipse is not made too wide, in order that direct closure of the skin edges may be achieved without use of a skin graft to bridge them.

The cosmetic result is reasonable (*Figure 14.3*), although the larger breasted the woman the more obvious the discrepancy. A range of silicone prostheses is available. In Nottingham a representative of a local stockist attends the breast cancer follow-up clinic each week to advise the patients. The prosthesis usually given is the Amoena Contour (Camp Ltd, Winchester). A nipple may be fitted over the prosthesis when summer dresses are worn.

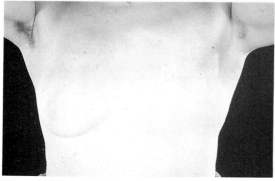

Figure 14.3 Patient who has undergone simple mastectomy

An excellent range of swimwear and of brassières is also available with pockets to contain the prosthesis: the range we use is from Anita Ltd (Donovan and Harrison, Shrewsbury).

The operation is straightforward, requiring a hospital stay of only 3–4 days, and physically has few sequellae. A degree of depression, most noticeable when the patient has just returned home from operation, and some anxiety are to be expected. These may be helped by counselling, which should be given by a specially trained counselling nurse. Sometimes the anxiety or depression may reach severe levels and treatment by a psychiatrist is required. The best arrangement is for one psychiatrist to look after such cases in any one health district and for the counselling nurse to liaise regularly with the psychiatrist and be able to seek help by direct reference. Perhaps up to 10 per cent of women with primary breast cancer require short-term psychiatric help, a larger number several visits and talks with the counselling nurse; only a very few require long-term help.

Reconstructive surgery

Many women who undergo mastectomy would like an operation which restores the breast or at least gives a cleavage and does not mean that they have to wear a prosthesis. This desire in our experience is, as one might expect, strongly age linked; younger women are often desperate at the thought of losing the breast. In the long term, women often adjust to their situation but levels of depression have been shown to be reduced by reconstructive surgery. Also this may not reflect the whole story and it is our experience that women who have had even an imperfect reconstruction are often pleased to have had this done.

The simplest method of reconstruction is to place a tissue expander under the skin or under the pectoral muscle. The tissue expander is inflated by saline injections of 50 ml/week, allowing the skin to gradually stretch. When an appropriate size is reached the expander is removed and a permanent silicone prosthesis replaces it. This method gives a 'mound' but without the nipple complex. The main complication is capsule formation around the prosthesis: a very tough fibrous capsule forms over several months and constricts the prosthesis, pushing it forwards in an unsightly fashion. This may require incising.

A better cosmetic result may be achieved by planning a subcutaneous mastectomy in the first

Breast conservation 71

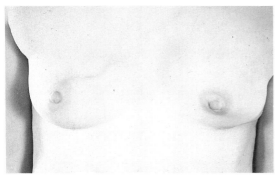

Figure 14.4 Patient 7 years after left subcutaneous mastectomy and silcone implant

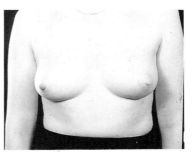

Figure 14.5 Patient with primary cancer treated by excision of the cancerous lump and whole breast irradiation

instance. In this operation, an incision is made in the inframammary fold and the breast tissue is dissected free of the underlying muscle and of the skin and subcutaneous fat, leaving the nipple and areola. In Nottingham we prefer to reconstruct 3 months later by reopening the wound and placing a silicone prosthesis subcutaneously. Again the prosthesis may be placed submuscularly which is said to carry a lower incidence of capsule formation.

The cosmetic result of this operation may be very good (*Figure 14.4*) and this is achieved in around a quarter of our patients. A further 50 per cent have an acceptable result (looks normal in a brassière and the patient does not have to wear any external prosthesis).

The operation is unsuitable if the tumour is near the nipple, as the nipple ducts will be involved, or if the patient has very large breasts. It is difficult to produce droop, although some is given by placing the prosthesis subcutaneously.

Breast conservation

The best cosmetic result is achieved by treating the cancer by excision of the lump followed by high dose radiotherapy to the whole breast. To ensure a good cosmetic result, the irradiation is given in a number of fractions (20–30 depending upon the centre), spread over 2–6 weeks. Cosmetic result is usually excellent (*Figure 14.5*) but the danger is recurrence of the cancer within the breast.

To minimize local recurrence, the tumour is taken with a margin of normal tissue around it and histological inspection of the margins of the excised tissue is undertaken. If this shows invasive cancer or carcinoma *in situ*, then a wider incision or even mastectomy is performed. The whole breast is treated with a radiation dose of 50 Gy and the site of excision receives a further boost; this is given either by external beam or by the implantation of iridium wires. The boost gives 15–20 Gy to the excision site.

Not all tumours are suitable for this type of treatment; many centres limit this therapy to tumours of 2 cm or less. We have found that tumours, which in any case carry a poor prognosis (poorly differentiated plus lymph node involvement), tend to recur and give uncontrolled local recurrence of the type seen in *Figure 14.6* in around 15 per cent and we are treating such tumours by mastectomy. Also there is a danger of recurrence in

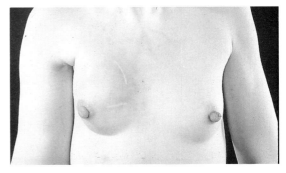

Figure 14.6 Uncontrolled local recurrence in patient with cancer previously treated by excision and irradiation

the breast when the surgical excision is microscopically incomplete. Multicentric tumours or breasts with widespread cancerous change may sometimes be detected preoperatively on mammography and are not suitable for this form of treatment. A preoperative mammogram is required for this reason (*Figure 14.7*) and also provides a base-line X-ray for follow-up mammograms to be compared with.

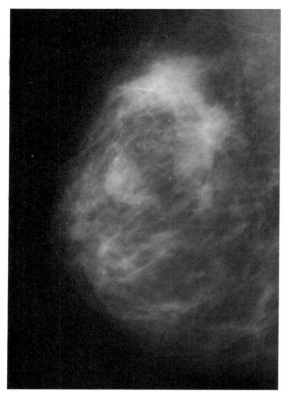

Figure 14.7 Mammogram shows widespread cancerous change in the breast although the palpable lump was small; this tumour is therefore not suitable for breast conservation by excision and whole breast irradiation

Choice of treatment

When a tumour is suitable for several methods of treatment, we advise the patient of the diagnosis, of the procedures available for treatment and of their disadvantages, e.g. breast conservation involves irradiation and a closer follow-up than mastectomy because of the danger of recurrence within the breast. Our counselling sister may take half an hour to an hour discussing this with the patient and her husband and helping the patient to choose her therapy. We have found that younger women invariably ask for breast conservation or reconstruction, older women for the simpler procedure of mastectomy.

The regional nodes

As discussed in Chapter 2, the primary route of spread of breast cancer is via the bloodstream.

Cancer also spreads through the lymphatics to the local lymph nodes. Once in the lymph nodes, the tumour may grow and give enlarged, painful glands. These may block the vein and lymphatics draining the arm and cause swelling of the arm.

If axillary nodes become enlarged with cancer they may be removed or treated by radiation. This is given as a dose of 45 Gy in 15 treatment sessions.

It used to be the fashion to use prophylactic irradiation following mastectomy. This may avoid having to treat the axilla at a later date. However, there are complications to irradiation, chiefly the lymphatics may become blocked and the arm swell or, most distressingly, the arm may become intensely painful from postirradiation inflammation of the nerves running from it. Only around 20 per cent of patients will require node irradiation subsequently if the nodes are initially left untreated. The Cancer Research Campaign trial which compared prophylactic irradiation with no treatment to the axillary nodes unless required during follow-up, showed that the latter policy was no less successful in avoiding uncontrolled growth in the axilla. Therefore prophylactic irradiation or prophylactic removal of the axillary nodes seems unnecessary.

Radical mastectomy

Radical mastectomy, described by Halstead in 1888, involves removal of the breast, the underlying pectoral muscles and the axillary glands up as far as the first rib. This procedure became the standard operation for breast cancer for many years and when X-ray therapy was introduced for cancer this was added to the operation. The cosmetic effect was unpleasant (although this was alleviated to some extent by the modified radical mastectomy introduced by Patey in 1938, which leaves the pectoralis major muscle) and there were a number of other side-effects.

Such radical treatments have been shown through a number of clinical trials to confer no benefit in terms of life expectancy over simple mastectomy.

Adjuvant systemic therapy

The measures described above control the tumour on the chest wall but do nothing for the secondary spread in distant organs that has already occurred.

As will be described in Chapter 16, when the secondary spread becomes apparent, hormonal therapy or chemotherapy may temporarily hold back the growth of the cancer. It seemed logical to try these agents as soon as possible, i.e. immediately following mastectomy, when the secondary spread is so often present but undetectable.

The results of trials studying the effect of this policy are now available and several results are apparent:

1. The use of either hormonal treatment (tamoxifen) or cytotoxic chemotherapy will delay the appearance of metastases in some patients.
2. There is a small improvement in survival at 5 years by either treatment.
3. Hormonal treatment seems the more effective in postmenopausal women and in fact adjuvant cytotoxic chemotherapy may only be working by halting ovarian activity in premenopausal women.
4. There are unpleasant side-effects from cytotoxic therapy.

It is our belief that we should first identify those patients unlikely to have trouble from secondary spread (*see* Chapter 1), e.g. well-differentiated primary tumours without lymph node invasion, and exclude these women from any adjuvant systemic therapy as they will do well anyway.

Postmenopausal women (who will suffer no side-effects from tamoxifen) in the other prognostic groups are then candidates for hormonal adjuvant therapy. Tamoxifen in premenopausal women gives menopausal effects and we prefer to reserve the treatment until treatment becomes necessary when secondary spread becomes symptomatic.

In Nottingham, we do not use cytotoxic therapy as an adjuvant because any benefit to a few women seems outweighed by the side-effects for the majority and because reserving these agents until the secondary spread is apparent is probably a better way to use them.

Locally advanced primary tumours

Women presenting with tumours over 5 cm in diameter (*see Figures 3.6* and *3.7*), which may be fixed deeply to the chest wall, have a very poor prognosis, only around 15 per cent being alive 5 years later. In addition the tumour is too large for mastectomy, which would often be followed by local recurrence.

The usual policy is to treat such tumours with radiotherapy (40 Gy in 15 fractions). We prefer to use tamoxifen (Nolvadex, ICI) 20 mg twice daily initially and watch the primary tumour. In hormone-responsive tumours (*see* Chapter 16), the primary will be controlled for some time and at the same time the tamoxifen is controlling the occult seconary spread in these tumours. When the tumour becomes unresponsive to hormone therapy, radiotherapy is given.

Breast cancer in the aged

'Old age' of course varies with the individual. In women really too old or unfit for mastectomy, we adopt a similar policy to that with locally advanced tumours.

Counselling

Around a quarter of all patients treated for primary breast cancer develop measurable levels of anxiety and/or depression and around a third will develop sexual problems; these patients can be identified and helped (*Figure 14.8*). The counselling nurse is involved in the care of the patient at an early stage – in fact at diagnosis in the clinic. In our unit the surgeon tells the patient the diagnosis and the counselling nurse is left with her to comfort her and then to meet her information needs about the treatment. This is especially important when a choice of treatments is possible, for example whether the patient would like breast conservation and its attendant risk of recurrence or would prefer mastectomy. If the patient wishes, her partner is involved at this stage.

Leaflets are given to her to reinforce what has been said explaining what will happen during her stay in hospital and any treatment that may follow, e.g. radiotherapy.

The patient is next seen by the counselling nurse on the ward the day before her operation; questions

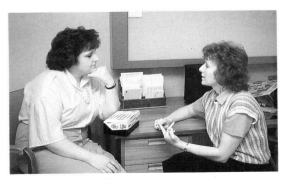

Figure 14.8 Counselling

are answered and discussion takes place about how the patient will come to terms with her disease and treatment.

Postoperatively the patient is visited, at home, by the counselling nurse; at this visit an assessment of her psychological state is carried out. Questions about her general health and mood are asked and her wound is checked. This gives the opportunity for questions about how she feels about the alteration in her body image, if her husband has seen her scar and if sexual problems are likely to develop.

If the counselling nurse believes that the patient has a high level of anxiety or depression then, by prior arrangement, she is directly referred for a psychiatric opinion from a psychiatrist who has taken a special interest in this problem. The counselling nurse is able to help the patient at future meetings with counselling, relaxation techniques and simple desensitizing techniques. The nurse must also check that the prosthesis is satisfactory and, if not, organize the provision of a new one. The patient is told to contact the nurse should problems arise and a card is given to her with a contact number.

Finally, with the advent of nation-wide breast screening, the role of the counselling nurse may well need to be extended to cover those patients recalled to the screening unit.

15

Radiology in the breast cancer follow-up clinic

In the follow-up clinic we watch for symptoms of metastatic spread and cancer of the opposite breast. Once a woman has undergone treatment for primary breast cancer, we follow her up by seeing her at 6-monthly intervals in our clinic. Any symptoms suggestive of secondary spread – back pain, breathlessness, severe loss of appetite and weight loss, headache – are investigated. The opposite breast and the mastectomy skin flaps, the axilla and, in cases of treatment by breast conservation, the treated breast are examined. The patient is told that the clinic is always open to her, should she be worried and wish to return between the regular appointments.

Bone scanning

Some clinicians start follow-up by carrying out a routine bone scan. Scanning is the most sensitive method of imaging metastatic carcinoma in bones; it may show lesions which would be invisible on bone X-ray. Because breast cancer most frequently spreads to bone, then scanning early in the course of the disease might seem a good idea. However, in several large series the detection rate of metastases by this method at the time of diagnosis of the primary tumour is only 1–2 per cent (*Table 15.1*). Also the only information the scan gives that we can act upon is that the cancer has spread – not just to the site imaged but to many other bones and to other organs. Knowledge of this is available to us from more accurate indices built on lymph node biopsy and from histological differentiation (*see* Chapter 1). Bone scanning at the time of diagnosis

Table 15.1 Results of bone scans in 354 patients at the time of treatment of the primary tumour

Result	Percentage (n = 354)
Positive	2.3
Negative	96.3
False positive	1.1
False negative	0.3

of the primary tumour is an expensive procedure giving us no extra information.

Bone scanning, however, definitely has its place in the follow-up clinic. At each visit the patient is asked about new or unusual aches or pains. Bone pain from distant metastases is most commonly a constant pain, bad enough to keep the patient awake and to make her take analgesics at all times. Any skeletal pain that cannot be easily dismissed is first investigated by a bone scan (*Figure 15.1*).

A scan is carried out using a technetium isotope ^{99}Tc-labelled polyphosphate. The phosphate is concentrated in areas of new bone formation, around arthritic areas or in the bone immediately surrounding bone metastases. The patient is given an intravenous injection of the polyphosphate and 2 hours later the scan is performed on a linear scanner or using a gamma camera.

The bone scan needs careful interpretation. A single 'hot spot' where the isotope is concentrated has to be examined by X-ray. It may prove to be non-malignant – patients who have received treatment for breast cancer are not immune from slipped discs! Pain, with a hot spot inexplicable by a benign

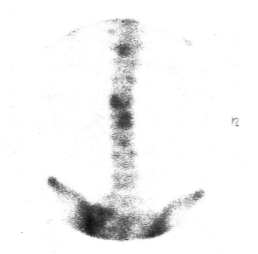

Figure 15.1 A bone scan carried out on a gamma camera. Hot spots, in this case indicative of metastases, are seen in the pelvis and the thoracic spine

cause, is considered to be due to a metastasis even if no metastasis is seen on the bone X-ray. Examples of metastases showing on X-ray are seen in *Figures 15.2* and *15.3*.

Bone X-rays

Where there is a danger that the bone may fracture from being weakened by a secondary deposit, then regular bone X-rays are required to assess whether orthopaedic stabilization is required (*see* Chapter 16).

Secondary deposits in the ribs are not uncommon, but occasionally a fracture of a rib is seen which is a side-effect of irradiation of the chest wall and not due to metastasis. This may occur a number of years after the treatment.

CT scans and MRI

Where there remains difficulty in diagnosing bone pain these techniques may be required (*Figure 15.4*).

Chest X-ray

Spread to the lungs may give symptoms of breathlessness or persistent cough. There are three

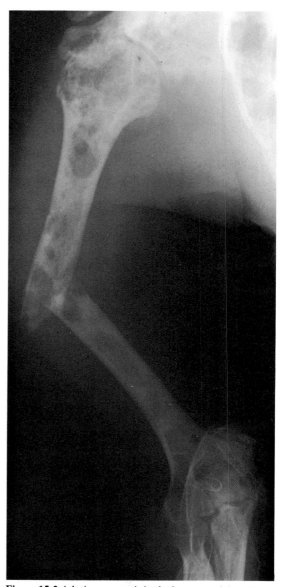

Figure 15.2 A lytic metastasis in the humerus giving rise to a fracture

X-ray presentations of lung metastases: pleural effusion where there are metastases on the lung surface irritating the pleura and producing fluid (*see Figure 1.3*), solid lung metastasis (*Figure 15.5*) and, most difficult to detect on X-ray, carcinomatous lymphangitis of the lungs (*Figure 15.6*) where the tumour has spread along the lymphatic vessels, widely permeating the lung.

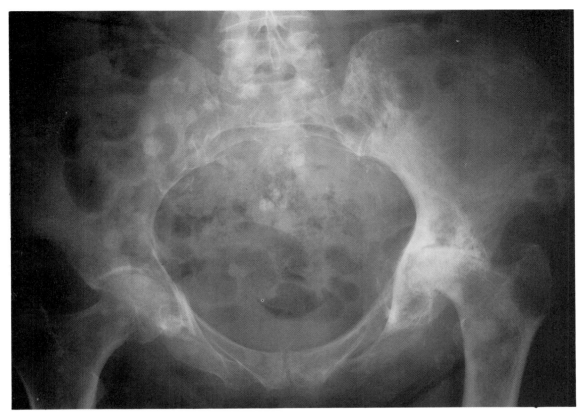

Figure 15.3 Blastic metastases (which are less common in breast cancer) in the pelvis

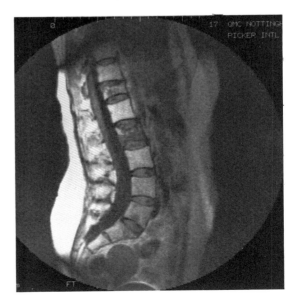

Figure 15.4 An MRI scan of the lumbar spine showing destruction of L3 and collapse of L1 from metastases from breast cancer

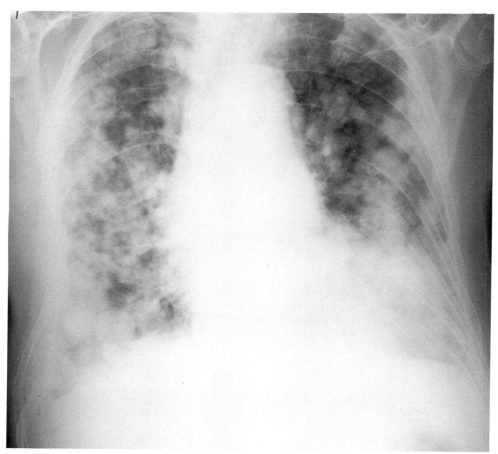

Figure 15.5 Chest X-ray showing multiple solid lung metastases

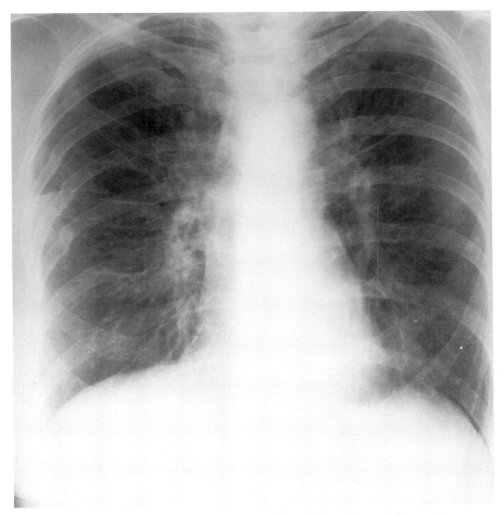

Figure 15.6 Chest X-ray showing carcinomatous lymphangitis. This is a widespread change with cancer growing down the lymphatic channels in the lung. It may be difficult to show on X-ray because the change is uniform all over the lung

Secondary spread to the liver

The patient may complain of severe lassitude, pronounced loss of appetite, weight loss and, if the liver is enlarged, pain in the upper abdomen.

The best confirmatory test is a rise in the serum alkaline phosphatase and the γ-glutamyl transferase. Imaging may be performed by isotope liver scans, ultrasound or CT scan (*Figure 15.7*), but in the presence of symptoms and disordered liver function tests these are an unnecessary extra expense.

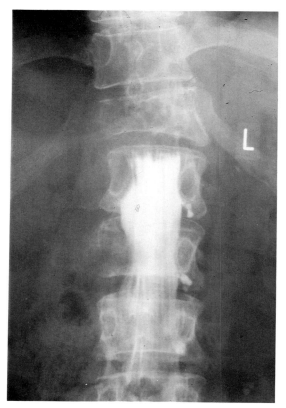

Figure 15.9 Myelogram showing a block in the subarachnoid space

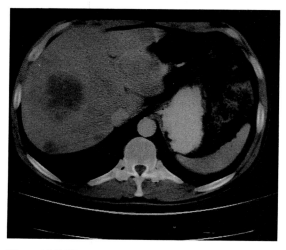

Figure 15.7 CT scan showing liver metastases

CNS metastases

Brain metastases may give rise to a variety of symptoms – severe headache, odd behaviour, incoordination, epilepsy and double vision. CNS metastases may also occur in the spinal cord giving weakness or paralysis below their level.

Brain metastases may be imaged by an isotope brain scan (*Figure 15.8*). This is carried out using ^{99m}Tc-labelled pertechnate. However, this technique has been superceded by CT scanning or by MRI, both of which have proved to be more accurate.

Metastases in the spinal cord (growing on the meningeal covering) are demonstrated by a myelogram (*Figure 15.9*), although again CT scanning or MRI are now non-invasive alternatives.

Mammography of the treated breast

Mammography in the follow-up clinic is used to follow breasts in which the cancers have been treated by excision and irradiation. Our routine here is to examine the brease clinically at 3-monthly

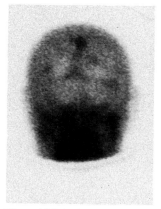

Figure 15.8 An isotope scan showing multiple filling defects in both hemispheres

intervals, with mammography at 6-monthly intervals, for 36 months. Thereafter clinical examination and mammography are carried out at 6-monthly intervals. Only the treated breast is imaged at each visit. Initially there is general oedema of the breast. This has largely settled by the 12-month follow-up.

Mammography of the opposite breast

A woman with a breast cancer has a 2 per cent chance of cancer in the opposite breast at the same time as the primary is diagnosed and thereafter a 1 per cent chance of opposite breast cancer per annum: this is 10 times the normal annual risk of contracting breast cancer.

Our policy is to carry out mammography at the time of treatment of the primary tumour in order to make sure there is not a detectable growth in the opposite breast.

During follow-up our approach to the opposite breast depends upon the patient's prognosis (*see* Chapter 1). There is little point in the early detection of a cancer of the opposite breast in a woman who is going to die of her initial breast cancer (poor prognostic group). In the other prognostic groups we carry out biennial single-view mammography of the opposite breast.

16

The treatment of advanced breast cancer

One woman in five undergoing mastectomy will be alive and free of metastases 20 years after operation (*see* Chapter 1), a number will die of natural causes before 20 years have passed, and the remainder (more than half) will show symptoms from metastatic spread (*see* Chapter 15). Once distant spread becomes symptomatic, the patient will die from her disease and two out of three will die within 2 years (*see Figure 1.4*).

Classification

Metastatic spread should be discussed under three main headings: local, regional and distant recurrence.

Local recurrence

This is the development of metastases in the mastectomy skin flaps. These may take the form of isolated 'spot' recurrences or they may be widely spread, often presenting as a dull, crimson, eczematous appearance – 'field change' due to a spread in dermal lymphatics (*Figure 16.1*).

Regional recurrence

This is the appearance of enlarged axillary or supraclavicular lymph nodes. Nodes may, of course, become enlarged for reasons other than spread of the carcinoma. Therefore, to make the diagnosis of regional recurrence it is better to suspect only large and hard nodes, and to confirm the diagnosis by needle biopsy or cytology.

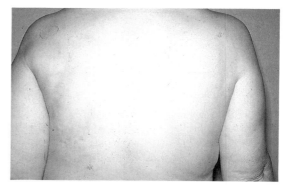

Figure 16.1 Widespread local recurrence in dermal lymphatics extending round to the back

Distant recurrence

This may present almost anywhere, but the commonest sites are bone, liver, lung and pleura. The diagnosis is not always straightforward and any woman who has undergone treatment for primary breast cancer should have a new symptom such as back pain fully investigated however many years afterwards. The symptoms and their radiological investigations are discussed in Chapter 15.

Treatment

Local recurrence

Isolated 'spot' recurrence is treated by excision. Multiple spot recurrence or 'field change' requires control by irradiation. However, the appearance of 'field change' is the herald of symptomatic distant metastases.

Regional recurrence

Regional recurrence may be treated by surgical clearance of the axilla or by irradiation. Once again, the appearance of rapidly enlarging cancerous nodes often indicates impending symptoms of distant spread.

Distant recurrence

The appearance of distant metastases means that systemic therapy must be implemented. However, local therapies also play a part depending upon the sites of metastases.

Local therapies

Bone

Irradiation should be used freely for bone metastases. This is especially indicated for painful bone metastases and for metastases in danger of collapse, for example vertebrae, the neck of the femur and the femoral shaft.

Impending or actual *fracture* of the femoral neck or shaft is treated by orthopaedic pin stabilization (*Figure 16.2*) plus irradiation. Where the vertebrae appear in danger of collapse, the clinician should be aware of possible paraplegia and should warn the patient to immediately report any symptoms. The breast cancer surgeon should have arrangements with the local neurosurgical centre for immediate

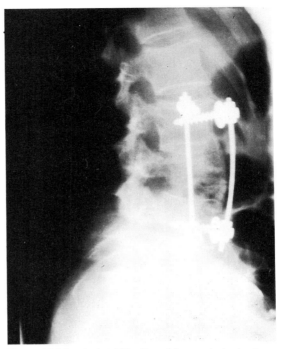

Figure 16.3 Surgical stabilization of the cervical spine to prevent quadriplegia

examination by a consultant neurologist or the rapid transfer to the centre of cases where there is even only suspicion of CNS motor changes. Surgical decompression within hours of a vertebral collapse with cord compression may prevent paraplegia (*Figure 16.3*).

Pleural effusion

A pleural effusion should be emptied by repeated aspiration or, if large, by an intercostal suction drain. Once the pleural cavity is empty of effusion, 40 ml containing tetracycline 1 g and 1% lignocaine is injected down the drain; this may be repeated if the effusion persists. Watch should be kept for the development of pericardial effusions.

Pulmonary carcinomatous lymphangitis

This gives severe dyspnoea. This is relieved to some extent by general measures: a broad-spectrum antibiotic to eliminate supra-added infection, prednisolone and aminophylline to eliminate any bronchospasm and using oxygen. Cytotoxic chemotherapy is used as the initial systemic therapy in carcinomatous lymphangitis.

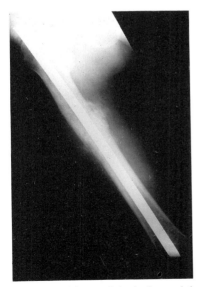

Figure 16.2 Metastasis in the femoral shaft stabilized by orthopaedic surgery

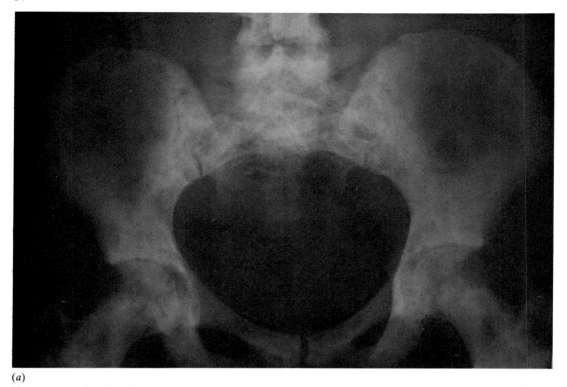

(a)

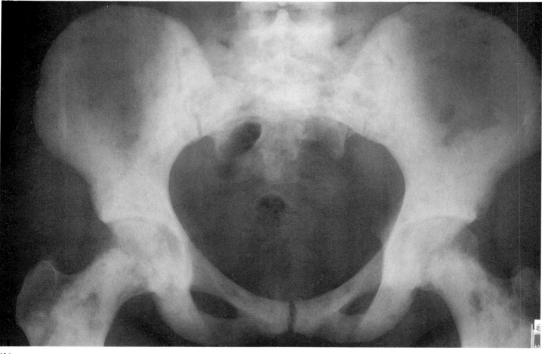

(b)

Figure 16.4 Lytic metastases in the pelvis before (a) and after (b) 6 months of treatment. Response to treatment is seen: the metastases have sclerosed

Brain metastases

These should be treated by systemic dexamethasone 4 mg 6-hourly in addition to the antitumorous systemic therapy. Brain metastases giving severe symptoms, such as headache, may be helped by irradiation.

Hypercalcaemia

This must be remembered or it is likely to take the clinician by surprise. The patient may present with the symptoms before bone metastases have been recognized. The symptoms are profound general malaise, weakness and nausea. The initial treatment is to ensure adequate hydration and to place the patient on systemic therapy against breast cancer. If this fails to restore the serum calcium to normal limits, then calcitonin or polyphosphates should be used.

Systemic therapy

Systemic therapy may be hormonal or by use of cytotoxic chemotherapy. On treatment the tumour deposits may apparently disappear altogether or get smaller (response) or stay static or progress on the treatment. At present radiology plays a considerable part in judging response. X-rays of selected bone metastases are taken at the start of treatment and are repeated at 2-monthly intervals. Response to therapy may be shown by diminution in size of the metastases or by sclerosis of a previously lytic metastasis (*Figure 16.4*). An increase in fat content of metastases on MRI appears to correlate with response to treatment.

The side-effects of many regimens of cytotoxic chemotherapy are unpleasant, while those of

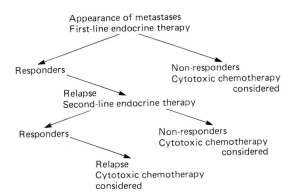

Figure 16.5 The overall plan for systemic therapy

hormonal manipulations may be negligible. Therefore the initial systemic therapy used is endocrinological. The overall plan is as shown in *Figure 16.5*.

Patients are assessed at 2 months from the start of, or any change in, therapy and then at 2-monthly intervals; those with obvious progression of disease are changed to a new treatment. They are then seen at 2-monthly intervals.

First-line endocrine therapy

Some breast cancers receive their drive from the circulating female hormones. Reducing the level of these or combating their effect may hold back the growth of breast cancer cells for a while – 3–4 years at the most. Premenopausal women until recently underwent oophorectomy whereas postmenopausal patients on our unit are given tamoxifen (Nolvadex, ICI) 20 mg twice daily. Tamoxifen acts by blocking the effect of circulating oestrogen on the cells. It is a drug with very few side-effects.

Recently a new drug, goserelin (Zoladex, ICI), has been investigated by our unit. It blocks the action of the ovaries and oophorectomy is now unnecessary. The premenopausal woman will probably receive both tamoxifen and goserelin in future. Side-effects of goserelin are again few, although the patient will of course have the effects of going through the menopause.

Second-line endocrine therapy

Those patients who respond to first-line endocrine therapy do so for an average of around 18 months. They then progress again and therapy has to be changed. Only those who responded to first-line endocrine therapy are given further endocrines: our choice is for megestrol acetate (Megace, Bristol-Myers; a progesterone) given in high dose (320 mg/day).

Prediction of response to endocrine therapy

The measurement of oestrogen receptor in tumour tissue raises the possibility of a biochemical measurement giving an absolute guide to whether the patient will respond to hormonal treatments or not. Thus, series reporting the results of response of metastases to first-line endocrine therapy compared with oestrogen receptor in the tumour, find a 40–50 per cent response in oestrogen receptor-positive tumours and 5–10 per cent response in oestrogen receptor negative. At present, however, the possible benefits of endocrine therapy, and the simplicity of first-line endocrine therapy, mean that this is usually employed first, even in oestrogen receptor-negative patients.

Cytotoxic chemotherapy

The success of regimens of cytotoxic chemotherapy in the lymphomas and leukaemias raised hopes of success in the treatment of solid cancers. Secondary breast cancer responds to combinations of chemotherapeutic drugs in 40–60 per cent of cases. However, response is short lived and the side-effects may be distressing: hair-loss, nausea, cystitis, sore mouth. Unfortunately, at present there are no means of determining which individual tumours are likely to respond to cytotoxic therapy.

Recently, less toxic drugs and regimens have been introduced such as mitozantrone (Lederle) or epirubicin (Farmitalia) in low dose. These regimens give few side-effects and enough patients show response or stabilization of disease to make their use worth while. These less toxic regimens have now become the drugs of choice after endocrine therapy.

Cytotoxic therapy should be introduced as the first line along with endocrine therapy for the patient breathless due to lung metastases.

Palliation and terminal care

It must be remembered that the responsibility of the team to the patient does not end when the tumour is no longer responsive to any form of therapy. The advice of a consultant specializing in pain control is a great aid and the patients may be admitted for short-term care in a number of circumstances, for example tapping effusions and controlling dyspnoea. Finally, access to hostel care for the terminal phase is invaluable when needed (*Figure 16.6*).

The initial efforts in pain relief should be directed at an overhaul of the drug schedule; this frequently results in excellent palliation. For example, bone pain may respond better to prostaglandin inhibitors than to the morphine derivates, and patients should be treated with indomethacin suppositories two twice daily and with frequent aspirin. As stated earlier, irradiation may give pain relief to bone metastases and should be employed where possible. The pain-relief consultant also has at his/her disposal slow-release morphine, local anaesthetic blocks, epidural morphine, hypnosis, acupuncture and the nerve cutting procedures of posterior rhizotomy, tractotomy and cordotomy.

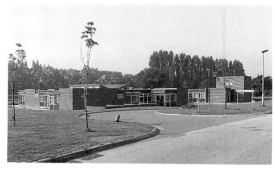

Figure 16.6 The pleasant situation on the Nottingham City Hospital Campus for Haywood House Continuing Care Centre

Specialist care for breast cancer

Although the various components of the care of the patient with breast cancer are each well within the scope of the appropriate consultant, the breast cancer patient is far better cared for by a team specializing in breast cancer. For example, the analysis of the X-rays to determine whether there is response to treatment is time consuming, and especially so for someone not used to carrying out this task. The dangers of staff in a number of disciplines separately looking after the patient is that none is responsible for formulating and following an overall plan for treatment of metastases. The team should include surgeon and radiotherapist, a specialist in pain relief, a pathologist well versed in breast cancer, a radiologist used to comparing sequential films of bone metastases and to reading bone scans, a counselling sister (in many ways the most important member of the team) and a psychiatrist used to problems of anxiety and depression in patients of this type. Needless to say, for the assessment of disease high quality X-rays and scans are required and these are the province of the radiographer.

The patient with metastases from breast cancer should therefore be cared for by a well-coordinated clinical team used to the problems. The team should work to a simple and predetermined treatment plan. The radiographer forms a part of this team in the imaging of metastases for diagnosis, treatment and for the very difficult tasks of the assessment of response to treatment. The patients are often ill and, with good reason, extremely anxious; a sensitive approach by the radiographer is a great bonus for the patient and a boost to the reputation of the team caring for her.

Appendix

Nottingham training programme for College of Radiographers recommended course

Radiographers attend a 3-day course (and also have some pre-course reading). Two days of the course are multidisciplinary with surgeons, radiologists and pathologists and include aspects of early detection and diagnosis and treatment of primary breast cancer, an introduction to pathology, radiology, radiographic techniques and the organization of a screening programme. The third day is a workshop day for radiographers only and covers physics of mammography and equipment testing with a physicist, quality control and quality assurance requirements with demonstrations and a full session on role play for radiographers in assessing clients' requirements and satisfaction, and the acquisition of counselling and communication skills.

Each radiographer attends the training unit for one week's secondment. The week includes an introduction to pattern recognition, a visit to an operating theatre, a ward round and one session in a busy GP referral breast clinic (a minimum of 50 mammograms under supervision). One session will be in the assessment clinic.

The radiographers have a log book in which to complete a further 250 mammograms to the satisfaction of the Training Centre. When this has been done a certificate of attendance is given which is logged at the College of Radiographers.

Index

Numbers given in italics refer to figures